TAPPING INTO FREEDOM

A Beginner's Guide to EFT Strategies for Stress, Anxiety, and Trauma. Steps for Daily Routines and Personalized Guidance to Improve Your Physical and Emotional Health

ELOISE ROSE

Copyright © Eloise Rose 2024 - All rights reserved.

The content contained within this book may not be reproduced, duplicated, or transmitted without direct written permission from the author or the publisher.

Under no circumstances will any blame or legal responsibility be held against the publisher, or author, for any damages, reparation, or monetary loss due to the information contained within this book. Either directly or indirectly. You are responsible for your own choices, actions, and results.

Legal Notice:

This book is copyright-protected. This book is only for personal use. You cannot amend, distribute, sell, use, quote, or paraphrase any part, or the content within this book, without the author's or publisher's consent.

Disclaimer Notice:

Please note the information contained within this document is for educational and entertainment purposes only. All effort has been executed to present accurate, up-to-date, and reliable, complete information. No warranties of any kind are declared or implied. Readers acknowledge that the author is not engaging in the rendering of legal, financial, medical, or professional advice. The content within this book has been derived from various sources. Please consult a licensed professional before attempting any techniques outlined in this book.

By reading this document, the reader agrees that under no circumstances is the author responsible for any losses, direct or indirect, which are incurred as a result of the use of the information contained within this document, including, but not limited to, — errors, omissions, or inaccuracies.

CONTENTS

Introduction	7
1. UNDERSTANDING EFT AND ITS FOUNDATIONS	11
1.1 What is EFT? An Introduction to Tapping	11
1.2 The Science Behind Tapping: How and Why It Works	13
1.3 The History of EFT: From Ancient Roots to Modern Practice	15
1.4 Understanding Meridian Points and Their Significance in EFT	17
2. PREPARING TO TAP: SETTING THE RIGHT FOUNDATION	21
2.1 Creating Your Personal Tapping Space: Environment Setup	21
2.2 Mental Preparation: Cultivating the Right Mindset for Tapping	24
2.3 Understanding and Setting Your Intentions for EFT	26
2.4 The Importance of Breathing Techniques in Tapping	28
3. STEP-BY-STEP TAPPING TECHNIQUES	31
3.1 Basic Tapping Sequence: A Step-by-Step Guide	31
3.2 Tapping for Daily Stress Relief: A Routine to Unwind	35
3.3 Quick Tapping Solutions for Sudden Anxiety	37
3.4 Integrating Affirmations with Your Tapping Practice	39
4. ADDRESSING EMOTIONAL CHALLENGES WITH EFT	43
4.1 Tapping Away Anxiety: Specific Techniques and Scripts	44
4.2 Overcoming Fear and Phobias with Targeted Tapping	46

    4.3 EFT for Managing Depression: A Gentle Approach — 48
    4.4 Healing Emotional Trauma through EFT — 50

5. TAPPING FOR PHYSICAL HEALTH — 55
    5.1 Using EFT to Alleviate Chronic Pain — 56
    5.2 EFT Techniques for Headache Relief — 58
    5.3 Tapping to Enhance Energy Levels — 60
    5.4 EFT for Digestive Health: A Holistic Approach — 62

6. ENHANCING SELF-CONFIDENCE AND PERSONAL GROWTH — 65
    6.1 Building Self-Esteem: Tapping into Your Potential — 66
    6.2 Overcoming Imposter Syndrome with EFT — 68
    6.3 Tapping for Public Speaking and Performance Anxiety — 71
    6.4 Using EFT to Set and Achieve Personal Goals — 73

7. SPECIALIZED TAPPING TECHNIQUES — 79
    7.1 Tapping for Emotional Eating and Weight Management — 79
    7.2 Advanced Tapping: Addressing Multiple Issues Simultaneously — 82
    7.3 Tapping Techniques for Relationship Issues — 85
    7.4 EFT for Professional and Workplace Stress — 87

8. INTEGRATING EFT INTO DAILY LIFE — 91
    8.1 Designing Your Daily Tapping Routine — 91
    8.2 Tapping While Traveling: Techniques on the Go — 94
    8.3 Incorporating Tapping into Morning and Evening Routines — 97
    8.4 Using Tapping to Maintain Emotional Balance Throughout the Day — 99

9. OVERCOMING COMMON CHALLENGES AND OBJECTIONS — 103
    9.1 "I Feel Silly Tapping": Overcoming Self-Consciousness — 104
    9.2 Dealing with Skepticism: How to Respond to Doubters — 105

    9.3 When Tapping Doesn't Work: Troubleshooting
    Common Issues   108
    9.4 Maintaining Motivation: What to Do When
    Progress Slows Down   110

10. SPECIAL POPULATIONS AND CONSIDERATIONS   113
    10.1 EFT for Children: Techniques and
    Considerations   113
    10.2 Tapping in Elderly Care: Adaptations and
    Benefits   116
    10.3 EFT for Athletes: Enhancing Performance and
    Recovery   118
    10.4 Cultural Considerations in the Practice of EFT   121

11. BEYOND TAPPING: COMPLEMENTARY
    PRACTICES   125
    11.1 Combining EFT with Meditation for Enhanced
    Calm   125
    11.2 Yoga and EFT: A Symbiotic Relationship for
    Healing   129
    11.3 Using Visualization Techniques Alongside
    Tapping   131
    11.4 The Role of Nutrition in Enhancing EFT
    Outcomes   133

12. CONTINUING YOUR JOURNEY WITH EFT   137
    12.1 Developing Your Own Tapping Scripts   137
    12.2 Staying Updated: Continuing Education in EFT   140
    12.3 Connecting with the EFT Community: Finding
    Support and Inspiration   142
    12.4 The Future of EFT: Trends and Innovations   144

    Conclusion   151
    References   153

INTRODUCTION

Six years ago, on a blustery spring morning, I found myself sitting on the edge of a neatly made hotel bed moments before a crucial business presentation. My heart and hands were pounding, and the room felt unbearably small. Panic gripped me, and no matter how much I tried to calm myself, nothing worked. Desperate, I remembered a technique a friend had mentioned – EFT or Emotional Freedom Techniques. Skeptical but cornered, I tried it. What happened next was nothing short of miraculous. Within minutes, my anxiety dissipated, replaced by a calm, focused energy I hadn't felt in years. That day, not only did I ace the presentation, but my life also took a new direction.

My journey into the world of EFT started quite unexpectedly. As a professional in the health and wellness industry, I was no stranger to various healing modalities, but EFT intrigued me with its simplicity and effectiveness. Over the years, I've seen firsthand how this powerful tool has transformed lives, including my own. From resolving deep-seated emotional issues to overcoming daily stresses, the impact of EFT has been profound and far-reaching.

This book is written for you, whether you're entirely new to EFT or are familiar with it but haven't yet experienced its full potential. I aim to demystify the process, giving you a step-by-step guide to its techniques and benefits. You'll find practical instructions, success stories, and a detailed exploration of integrating these practices into your daily life.

You might be someone struggling with anxiety, eager to heal old wounds, or simply looking for ways to live a more empowered, confident life. Whatever your reason, this book promises to be a compassionate guide, offering you the tools you need for personal transformation.

This book's style is straightforward and empathetic. I understand the challenges of learning something new, especially as personal as tapping into your emotional processes. Therefore, this book is designed to be as accessible and supportive as possible, explaining complex concepts in clear, everyday language.

Unlike other texts on EFT, this book combines the latest research with practical applications and personal stories to give you a holistic understanding of the practice. You'll learn the 'how' and the 'why,' focusing on making EFT relatable and adaptable to your circumstances. We'll cover everything from the basics of tapping to specific strategies for different issues, ensuring you have a comprehensive toolkit at your disposal.

This book is structured to gradually build your knowledge and confidence. Starting with the foundational principles of EFT, we'll move through specific techniques for addressing emotional and physical ailments, enhancing personal growth, and finally, ways to incorporate tapping into your daily routines. Each chapter builds on the last, progressively allowing you to develop your skills.

Transform your life with EFT: By the end of this book, you will thoroughly understand EFT and how it can help you. You'll also be equipped with practical tools to implement this powerful technique, paving the way for significant personal change.

CHAPTER 1

UNDERSTANDING EFT AND ITS FOUNDATIONS

Have you ever felt a sudden, overwhelming sense of calm after a simple act like rubbing your temples or taking a deep breath? This automatic response to touch and pressure is deeply rooted in human physiology, hinting at body-focused practices' broader, untapped potential to heal and restore us. Emotional Freedom Techniques, or EFT, leverage this innate power through a structured approach to tapping on specific body points, marrying the age-old wisdom of acupressure with the insights of modern psychology. This chapter aims to peel back the layers of EFT, offering you a clear and thorough understanding of its mechanisms, components, and profound capacity for healing.

1.1 WHAT IS EFT? AN INTRODUCTION TO TAPPING

EFT, commonly known as tapping, is a psychological acupressure technique gaining recognition due to its simplicity and effectiveness in treating various physical and emotional issues. At its core, EFT combines elements of traditional Chinese medicine—specifically, the concept of meridians or energy pathways within the body—with cognitive psychology. The technique involves tapping with the fingertips on specific meridian points while focusing on negative emotions or physical sensations. This dual engagement of somatic and cognitive focus aims to release energy blockages believed to be the root cause of emotional distress and physical ailments.

The basic mechanics of tapping are straightforward yet powerful. By gently tapping on specific points on the body, you can influence the body's energy system. These points include areas around the eyebrows, the sides of the eyes, under the eyes, under the nose, the chin, the beginning of the collarbone, and under the arms. Each of these points corresponds to different physical and emotional aspects of well-being. The physical act of tapping is combined with vocalizations of specific issues or affirmations, which helps to center the mind on particular problems or thoughts. This combination works to balance the energy system, which can reduce physical and emotional pain.

An EFT session typically consists of three main components: the Setup Statement, the Tapping Sequence, and the Reflection Phase. The Setup Statement is designed to acknowledge the issue and accept oneself despite the problem. It usually starts with the phrase, "Even though I have this [fear, pain, problem], I deeply and completely accept myself." This is followed by the Tapping Sequence, where you tap on the specific points in a particular order while repeating a reminder phrase related to the issue. The session ends with the Reflection Phase, where you take a moment to sit quietly and pay attention to the feelings and thoughts that arise, assessing any shift in intensity of the original emotion or pain.

The benefits and goals of EFT are widespread, addressing issues from anxiety and depression to physical pain and performance enhancement. The tapping process calms the nervous system, rewires the brain to respond healthier, and promotes a more profound sense of overall well-being. People who use EFT often report feeling lighter, more empowered, and less burdened by their emotional and physical ailments.

Interactive Element: Quick Self-Assessment

Here's a quick self-assessment exercise to help you connect more personally with the information provided. Reflect on a recent situation where you experienced significant stress or discomfort. Ask yourself:

- What physical sensations did you notice?
- What emotions were you feeling?
- On a scale of 1-10, how intense was the experience?

Jot these down in a journal or note-taking app. As you learn more about EFT in the following sections, you'll have the opportunity to apply tapping techniques to this specific experience, allowing you to feel the effects of EFT on your issues directly.

1.2 THE SCIENCE BEHIND TAPPING: HOW AND WHY IT WORKS

In exploring the scientific foundation of EFT, it's crucial to acknowledge the research that underscores its effectiveness, particularly in reducing cortisol levels and mitigating stress and anxiety. Several studies have documented the physiological impacts of EFT, offering a compelling argument for its use as a therapeutic technique. For instance, a significant study published in the *Journal of Nervous and Mental Disease* reported that EFT lowered cortisol levels and symptoms of psychological distress in participants significantly more than other interventions. Cortisol, often called the "stress hormone," plays a critical role in various body functions, and its reduction is closely linked to a decrease in overall stress levels.

The mechanisms behind EFT extend beyond simple relaxation, delving into the cognitive shifts that occur during tapping. When engaging in EFT, individuals focus on a specific negative emotion or issue while tapping on meridian points. This process has been shown to create a balance in the energy system, often disrupted by stress or trauma. Focusing on a negative issue while engaging in a physical action that promotes calm can lead to cognitive shifts. Essentially, the brain associates the previously distressing thought with a new, calmer bodily response. This phenomenon is akin to 'rewiring' the brain's conditioned responses, making EFT a potent tool for addressing deep-seated emotional disturbances.

Physiologically, EFT has been shown to influence several areas of the body directly involved in the stress response. One of the primary regions affected is the amygdala, often called the brain's fear center. Studies using fMRI scans have shown that tapping can reduce amygdala activity, alleviating stress and anxiety. Furthermore, EFT has been observed to alter brain wave patterns, promoting a state more conducive to relaxation and healing. These changes are not merely subjective; they represent measurable neurological shifts that enhance our understanding of how EFT facilitates emotional and physical healing.

Despite its growing popularity and the positive outcomes reported in numerous studies, EFT has faced skepticism from some quarters of the scientific community. Critics often question the methodology of studies and the theoretical basis of meridian systems used in tapping. However, this skepticism has also fueled more rigorous investigations into EFT, leading to better-designed studies that strengthen the case for its effectiveness. Both practitioners and clients need to consider these critiques and counterpoints as they encourage ongoing dialogue and research that ultimately enhance the practice and understanding of EFT.

In practical terms, the growing body of research and the continued scrutiny of EFT contribute to its evolution as a respected therapeutic practice. As more studies are conducted and published, understanding how tapping affects the brain and body deepens, providing valuable insights for those who practice and rely on EFT to relieve psychological and physiological symptoms. This ongoing cycle of research and application fosters a more profound comprehension and broader acceptance of EFT as a legitimate tool in psychological health and well-being.

1.3 THE HISTORY OF EFT: FROM ANCIENT ROOTS TO MODERN PRACTICE

The story of Emotional Freedom Techniques (EFT) is a fascinating journey through time, bridging ancient healing principles with contemporary therapeutic practices. The roots of EFT trace back to the ancient Chinese meridian system, a cornerstone of traditional Chinese medicine. This system posits that the human body is traversed by a network of pathways or meridians through which life energy, or 'Qi,' flows. These pathways connect to specific organs and functions, and disruptions in this energy flow are believed to cause disease and emotional distress. The practice of acupuncture, which involves inserting needles into specific points along these meridians to rebalance the flow of Qi, is a well-known application of this theory. In a modern twist, EFT also taps into this ancient wisdom using fingertip tapping rather than needles, targeting similar meridian points to restore balance and promote healing.

The development of EFT as we know it today began with a significant breakthrough by Dr. Roger Callahan in the 1980s. His creation, Thought Field Therapy (TFT), was the precursor to EFT and represented a radical new approach to treating emotional distress. Callahan discovered tapping on specific meridian points could alleviate emotional disturbances, which came about serendipitously. While working with a patient with a severe phobia of water, Callahan, guided by his knowledge of the meridian system, asked her to tap an endpoint of the stomach meridian under her eye. To his astonishment, her phobia was immediately relieved. This incident sparked a deeper exploration into the relationship between the body's energy systems and emotional health, leading to the development of TFT.

EFT was later developed by Gary Craig, a Stanford engineering graduate and a student of Callahan's. Craig believed that the benefits of tapping could be accessible to a much wider audience and set about simplifying the complexity of Thought Field Therapy. He introduced a streamlined approach that reduced the need for complex diagnostic procedures to identify the correct tapping points. Instead, Craig proposed a comprehensive tapping routine encompassing all primary meridian endpoints, reasoning that this would cover all necessary bases without requiring intricate customization. This democratization of the technique significantly broadened its appeal and usability, leading to the widespread adoption of EFT.

Since its inception, EFT has evolved and expanded in its scope and application, transcending its initial focus on phobias and emotional distress. Today, EFT is used worldwide to address a broad array of psychological and physical issues, from anxiety and depression to chronic pain and performance enhancement. Its efficacy and ease of use have garnered a large following among therapists and individuals seeking a powerful self-help tool that can be practiced independently or in conjunction with other therapeutic treatments.

The evolution of EFT has been shaped significantly by critical figures whose work has helped to refine and validate the practice. Beyond Gary Craig, numerous practitioners and researchers have contributed to the growth and legitimation of EFT. These include individuals like Dr. Dawson Church, whose research into the physiological effects of EFT has provided valuable scientific backing, and Dr. David Feinstein, a clinical psychologist who has been instrumental in exploring and documenting the mechanisms through which EFT affects the brain and body. Their contributions, along with those of many others in the field, have been crucial in establishing EFT as a respected and effective therapeutic modality.

Today, EFT stands as a testament to the enduring wisdom of ancient healing practices and the innovative application of modern psychological principles. As it continues to evolve, the EFT journey remains a compelling example of how the past and present can converge to create powerful new tools for healing and growth. EFT's ongoing development and application in various health and wellness fields highlight its versatility and potential to profoundly enhance human well-being.

1.4 UNDERSTANDING MERIDIAN POINTS AND THEIR SIGNIFICANCE IN EFT

Central to the practice of EFT, Meridian points are specific areas of the human body that are energetically connected to particular organs and emotional states through meridian pathways. These pathways, fundamental to traditional Chinese medicine (TCM), are thought to be channels through which the life force or 'Qi' flows. This concept, while ancient, is the cornerstone upon which EFT builds its methodology. In the realm of EFT, tapping on these meridian points while focusing on emotional disturbances is believed to release blockages in these energy channels, facilitating healing and restoring balance.

In TCM, each meridian is associated with an organ system and emotions. For instance, the lung meridian is often linked to sadness and grief, while the liver meridian correlates with anger and frustration. Tapping specific points along these meridians can alleviate the emotional burdens tied to these pathways when applying EFT. For example, tapping on the points around the eyes, which connect with the bladder meridian, may help relieve emotional stress that manifests physically, often in headaches or eye strain. Similarly, tapping the side of the hand, associated with the small intestine meridian, can help manage digestive disturbances alongside feelings of anxiety or defensiveness, echoing the interconnectedness of emotional and physical health.

The scientific community, traditionally skeptical about the concepts of TCM, has begun exploring the physiological implications of meridian points and their role in healing. Contemporary research has shown intriguing results while still nascent compared to more established medical sciences. Studies involving technologies like infrared imaging and electrical conductivity devices have observed measurable changes in the body's electrical field at these points, suggesting a physiological basis for what TCM has long posited about the existence and significance of meridians. These studies hint at the meridian points being areas of lowered electrical resistance and suggest that these points, when stimulated through methods like acupuncture or tapping, can influence the body's bioelectric field, potentially impacting various physiological processes.

Mapping these points to specific emotional relief is a nuanced aspect of EFT, rooted deeply in understanding each point's physical location and emotional significance. For instance, the point at the eyebrow's beginning is traditionally associated with being stuck or overwhelmed. When individuals tap on this point while vocalizing their specific emotional stress, they often find a decrease in the intensity of their feelings. This process, which involves tapping through a sequence that covers all primary meridian endpoints, ensures that the practitioner addresses a comprehensive range of emotional and physical issues.

Diagrams and illustrations of meridian points play a pivotal role in this process. These visual aids help practitioners and newcomers locate these points accurately and serve as educational tools, enhancing the understanding of how these points are interconnected across the body. Visual representations often include lines connecting the points, mirroring the meridians' descriptions in traditional Chinese diagrams, thus providing a clear map for both tapping sequences and understanding how energy flows through the body. These diagrams ensure that EFT practice is accessible and practical, allowing individuals to apply the technique with greater precision and confidence.

In practice, the application of EFT and the stimulation of these meridian points can be profoundly transformative. Consider the example of someone dealing with chronic stress, a condition notoriously tricky to manage and fraught with both physical and emotional ramifications. By using EFT, tapping on points like those along the heart or splay meridian, often associated with anxiety and worry, this individual can experience temporary relief and usually a profound shift in their overall stress response. Such results validate the significance of these points and underscore the potential of tapping to serve as a powerful tool for self-regulated healing.

Integrating this knowledge into practices like EFT broadens the scope of self-help methodologies as we continue to explore and validate the functions and benefits of meridian points through traditional practices and modern scientific inquiry. It enriches our understanding of the human body's complex and intricate nature. Blending ancient wisdom with contemporary science exemplifies holistic health practices' dynamic and evolving landscape, offering promising avenues for personal health management and therapeutic advancements.

CHAPTER 2

PREPARING TO TAP: SETTING THE RIGHT FOUNDATION

Imagine stepping into a serene garden, where the gentle sound of leaves rustling and a distant trickle of water are the only sounds. Each step deepens your sense of calm, preparing you to embrace a moment of healing and reflection. Just as this garden provides an ideal setting for tranquility, creating a personal space for your Emotional Freedom Techniques (EFT) practice plays a crucial role in enhancing the effectiveness of each session. This chapter guides you through establishing a physical and symbolic environment that supports your journey through EFT, ensuring that each tapping session is as beneficial as possible.

2.1 CREATING YOUR PERSONAL TAPPING SPACE: ENVIRONMENT SETUP

Choosing a Quiet and Comfortable Location

The first step in your EFT practice is selecting an appropriate space. This space doesn't need to be large or elaborately decorated;

it simply needs to be a place where you can find peace and privacy. Ideal locations include a seldom-used corner of your bedroom, a dedicated nook in your study, or even a quiet spot on your back porch. The key is consistency and comfort—choose a place where you can sit or stand comfortably and to which you can return regularly. This consistency helps to build a mental association between the space and the calming effects of EFT, making it easier over time to slip into a relaxed state as soon as you enter this space.

Setting Up the Physical Space

Once you have chosen your location, consider how to make it conducive to relaxation and focus. Start with comfortable seating; a chair that supports your back or even a cushion on the floor can work well. Add elements that soothe the senses - a soft blanket, calming colors, or a piece of art that evokes peace. Incorporating elements of nature, such as plants, a small fountain, or a window with a view of the garden, can enhance the calming effect of your environment. These elements of nature are not just decorative; they promote relaxation and reduce stress, making them perfect complements to your EFT practice.

Importance of Privacy

Privacy is crucial in EFT practice as it involves expressing and processing personal and sometimes sensitive emotions. Finding privacy in shared living spaces can be challenging but possible. Consider sessions early in the morning or late at night when others are less likely to interrupt. Alternatively, use subtle sound barriers like a white noise machine or soft background music to create a sense of seclusion. Communicating with the people you live with about the importance of this time and space can also help them respect your privacy.

Creating a Ritual

A simple ritual can significantly enhance your tapping practice by signaling to your brain that it is time to shift focus from the external to the internal. This ritual could be as simple as lighting a candle, arranging your space, or playing a particular music that soothes you. Setting up your space this way can be meditative, helping you transition into a more mindful state conducive to effective tapping. Over time, this ritual will become a powerful cue, preparing your mind and body to engage fully with the EFT process.

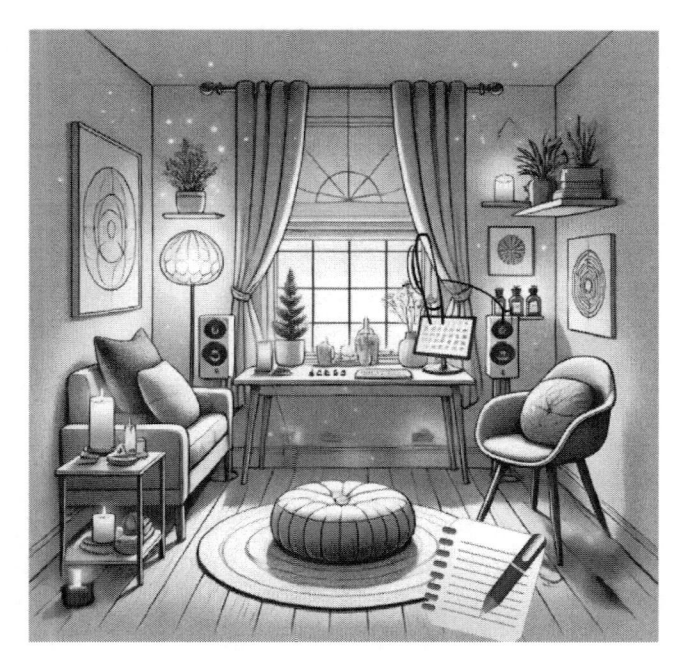

Create your own space

By thoughtfully setting up your tapping space, you create a sanctuary for emotional and physical healing. This environment, tailored to your personal comfort and privacy needs, becomes a crucial ally in your EFT practice, supporting you in exploring and releasing the emotional energies that impact your well-being. As you continue to refine this space and your approach to EFT, you'll find it becoming a powerful tool in your journey toward personal growth and healing.

2.2 MENTAL PREPARATION: CULTIVATING THE RIGHT MINDSET FOR TAPPING

Approaching Emotional Freedom Techniques (EFT) with an open mind and a heart full of acceptance is beneficial and essential. Imagine EFT as a seed you plant in the fertile soil of your consciousness. Just as a seed needs the right environment to germinate, your mindset plays a crucial role in nurturing and unleashing the potential benefits of EFT. Cultivating openness means exploring and accepting your emotions and experiences without judgment. This attitude sets a foundation where healing and profound change can occur. Tapping while harboring skepticism or resistance is akin to planting that seed in barren soil. It might grow, but the process will be stunted and more challenging.

The effectiveness of your tapping sessions is significantly influenced by your ability to accept yourself and the process. Acceptance here means acknowledging your feelings and experiences without attempting to force change or immediately remedy your discomfort. This might feel counterintuitive, especially if you're dealing with painful emotions. However, the acceptance stage is crucial because it allows you to approach your issues with compassion rather than criticism. When you start tapping, you're conversing with yourself, exploring areas of your psyche that need care and understanding. If this conversation begins with acceptance, the subsequent healing steps can proceed more smoothly and effectively.

Skepticism is a natural initial response for many beginners, especially those accustomed to more traditional therapy and medicine. If you are doubting, consider maintaining a journal dedicated to your EFT sessions. In this journal, record your feelings before and after each session, noting any shifts or insights. This record can serve as tangible evidence of the changes occurring, however subtle they may be initially. Over time, reviewing this journal can help solidify your understanding of EFTs impact and validate the process, gradually eroding skepticism.

Setting realistic expectations is another cornerstone of mental preparation for EFT. It's important to understand that while EFT has been profoundly transformative for many, its effects can vary widely among individuals. Factors such as personal history, the intensity of the issue, and individual emotional resilience play roles in how one experiences the outcomes of tapping. Some might find relief after a few sessions, while others may need a more extended period to notice significant changes. Adjusting your expectations to embrace this variability helps mitigate frustration and encourages a more patient, gentle approach to your healing process.

Lastly, preparing mentally to face potentially distressing emotions during tapping sessions is pivotal. EFT often brings deep-seated and sometimes painful feelings to the surface. Preparing yourself to encounter these emotions involves fostering a mindset of self-compassion and resilience. Remind yourself that it's okay to feel uncomfortable or emotional during tapping. These reactions are normal and indicative of the process working, of you reaching areas that need healing. To support yourself, you might establish safety mechanisms before you begin, such as setting aside time after sessions to engage in comforting activities or having a supportive person to talk to about your experiences. This preparation ensures that you are not overwhelmed and can conduct your tapping sessions within a safe, controlled context, allowing for emotional processing and healing to occur in a supportive environment.

2.3 UNDERSTANDING AND SETTING YOUR INTENTIONS FOR EFT

One of the most pivotal aspects of mastering Emotional Freedom Techniques (EFT) lies in setting clear and purposeful intentions before each session. Think of intentions as your roadmap; without them, you could still move forward, but with them, your journey becomes more directed and meaningful. Setting intentions helps you pinpoint exactly what you want to achieve through EFT, whether alleviating specific anxiety symptoms, enhancing your sleep quality, or perhaps fostering a more profound sense of self-compassion. By defining these goals clearly, you give direction to your tapping sessions and empower yourself to monitor your progress and celebrate your successes along the way.

The process of establishing clear goals begins with reflection. Take a moment to consider what you truly seek to change or achieve. It might help to ask yourself questions like, "What aspect of my life feels unbalanced?" or "What emotions am I finding overwhelming?" Answers to these inquiries can guide you toward creating focused and actionable objectives. For example, if you notice a recurring pattern of stress leading up to work presentations, your EFT goal might be to reduce performance anxiety and increase confidence in public speaking settings.

The significance of setting intentions extends beyond mere goal-setting; it actively enhances the effectiveness of your tapping sessions. When you tap with a clear intention, each action and each phrase used is infused with purpose, making your sessions more targeted and potent. This focused energy helps to align your subconscious mind with your conscious goals and amplifies the emotional and energetic work done during each tapping sequence. As you tap on the meridian points, you're not just going through the motions; you're actively engaging with and working to transform specific aspects of your life.

Aligning your EFT practice with your broader life values and goals enriches the experience and embeds it more deeply into your daily life, enhancing overall congruence. For example, suppose one of your core values is to lead a peaceful and harmonious life, and you find yourself frequently upset by minor inconveniences. In that case, you might set an intention to use EFT to cultivate greater emotional resilience and calmness. This alignment ensures that your EFT practice addresses specific issues and supports your larger life aspirations, making the benefits of tapping both profound and far-reaching.

Visualization is a powerful tool that can be employed to enhance the intention-setting process. Visualizing the desired outcomes as part of setting your intentions can prime your mind and body for positive change, creating a mental and emotional blueprint that guides your tapping practice. For instance, if you intend to reduce anxiety, you might visualize yourself handling a previously stressful situation calmly and efficiently. This mental imagery sets a positive expectation, which your mind and body can begin to work towards as you tap. Engaging in this visualization regularly as part of your EFT routine can significantly strengthen your focus and reinforce the manifestation of your goals, making the imagined outcomes more attainable.

By defining clear goals, aligning them with your values, and enhancing them through visualization, you create a robust framework for your EFT sessions that ensures each tapping sequence is as effective and transformative as possible. This deliberate and thoughtful approach to setting intentions not only maximizes the benefits you derive from EFT but also deeply personalizes the practice, making it an integral part of your emotional and physical well-being journey. As you refine and adapt your intentions based on your evolving needs and insights, your EFT practice remains dynamic and responsive, effectively supporting you in achieving temporary relief and sustained growth and healing.

2.4 THE IMPORTANCE OF BREATHING TECHNIQUES IN TAPPING

Breathing, as natural as it is vital, is key to enhancing the effectiveness of your Emotional Freedom Techniques (EFT) sessions. When you learn to control your breath, you gain a direct pathway to calming the nervous system, which is essential in preparing both mind and body for the emotional and physical release that tapping can facilitate. Controlled breathing helps reduce stress and ensures that your body is optimally prepared to engage in the EFT process. By focusing on your breath, you can lower your heart rate and blood pressure, creating a state of calm that makes it easier to address deep-seated emotions during tapping.

Integrating breathing techniques into your EFT sessions enhances the tapping experience significantly. Begin by incorporating deep breathing into the setup statement of your tapping routine. As you state your affirmation—acknowledging and accepting your feelings about the issue—take slow, deep breaths. Inhale deeply through your nose, allowing your abdomen to expand fully, and then exhale slowly through your mouth. This type of breathing encourages maximum oxygen exchange and triggers a relaxation response in the brain. Here's a step-by-step guide to integrating deep breathing with your tapping routine:

1. Find a Comfortable Position: Sit or stand in a comfortable position where you feel your body supported.
2. Start with the Setup Statement: As you begin reciting your setup statement, place one hand on your chest and the other on your abdomen. This will help you become more aware of your breathing pattern.
3. Inhale Slowly: Inhale slowly through your nose, focusing on filling your abdomen with air rather than your chest.
4. Exhale Gradually: While tapping on the first meridian point, slowly exhale through your mouth, releasing the air and any tension you might feel.
5. Continue Through Tapping Points: Maintain this breathing pattern as you move through the tapping points, allowing your breath to guide the rhythm of your tapping.

Exploring different breathing techniques can further tailor your EFT experience to your needs. Belly breathing, for example, is particularly effective for reducing anxiety and stress. It involves breathing deeply into the belly rather than the chest and is known for quickly calming the nervous system. The 4-7-8 breathing technique, another helpful method, involves breathing in for 4 seconds, holding the breath for 7 seconds, and exhaling for 8 seconds. This technique is beneficial in reducing anxiety and helping with sleep disturbances, which can be particularly useful if you're using EFT to manage insomnia or stress-related issues. Alternate breathing, often used in yoga, involves closing one nostril while breathing through the other and switching. This method helps balance the brain's left and right hemispheres, promoting mental clarity and emotional balance.

Regular breathing techniques can significantly enhance their effectiveness even outside your EFT sessions. By incorporating breathing exercises into your daily routine, you build a habit that supports your tapping and contributes to overall emotional resilience. You might start with a few minutes each morning, using deep breathing to set a calm tone for the day, or use 4-7-8 breathing before bed to ensure a restful night's sleep. The more you practice, the more natural these breathing techniques will feel, making them more effective when integrated into your tapping sessions.

By strategically using breathing techniques, you enhance your control over your body's stress response, making each EFT session more focused and effective. The ability to calm the nervous system on demand is a powerful tool for EFT, managing daily stresses and enhancing overall well-being. As you become more adept at using your breath in conjunction with tapping, you'll find that each session becomes a more profound, more transformative experience, allowing you to address specific issues and support a broader journey towards health and balance.

As this chapter concludes, we acknowledge the profound impact that a well-prepared environment, mindset, and intentional breathing can have on enhancing the effectiveness of EFT. These foundational elements set the stage for a tapping practice that is not only therapeutic but transformative, aligning deeply with your personal goals and values. As we transition into the next chapter, we'll explore specific tapping techniques in detail, building on the solid foundation you've established through thoughtful preparation. This progression ensures you have the knowledge and practical skills to apply EFT effectively, supporting your emotional freedom and resilience journey.

CHAPTER 3

STEP-BY-STEP TAPPING TECHNIQUES

Imagine you've just discovered a hidden switch inside you that could instantly ease your anxiety, soothe your stress, and transform your day from overwhelming to manageable. This isn't just a fantasy—it's the potential reality of mastering the primary tapping sequence in Emotional Freedom Techniques (EFT). This chapter is your guide to unlocking this powerful tool. Each tap can bring you closer to emotional freedom and personal empowerment as you learn to navigate the landscape of your body's energy points with precision and intention.

3.1 BASIC TAPPING SEQUENCE: A STEP-BY-STEP GUIDE

Understanding the Sequence

The journey into the world of EFT begins with mastering the primary tapping sequence, a cornerstone of effective practice. This sequence is a carefully structured approach that involves several key steps: identifying the problem, articulating the problem, measuring the intensity of the emotional or physical discomfort, and performing the tapping sequence on each designated point.

To start, clearly identify the issue you wish to address. It could be anything from a specific fear or anxiety to physical pain or a general feeling of unease. The more precise you are about what you want to tackle, the more effective your tapping will be. Next, articulate this problem. Put it into words that resonate with your feelings, which might require some introspection. This articulation is crucial as it directs your mind and energy toward the specific problem during the tapping process.

Once the issue is identified and articulated, measure the intensity of your feelings on a scale from 0 to 10, with 10 being the most intense. This initial measurement is essential as it provides a baseline to compare against after you complete your tapping sequence, allowing you to gauge the session's effectiveness.

Detailed Point Guide

Each tapping point in the sequence corresponds to a meridian point traditionally used in Chinese medicine, believed to be areas where energy channels converge. Here's a detailed walkthrough of each point:

1. Top of the Head (TOH): This point is right at the crown of your head. Tapping here influences the entire system and is an excellent place to start and finish the sequence.
2. Eyebrow (EB): Located at the beginning of the eyebrow, just above and to one side of the nose. This point is associated with managing stress and anxiety.
3. Side of the Eye (SE): This is on the bone bordering the outside corner of the eye and is linked with clarity of thought and vision.

4. Under the Eye (UE): Found under the eye, on the bone directly below your pupil when you're looking straight ahead. It's connected to easing sadness and fear.
5. Under the Nose (UN): The area between the nose and the upper lip. This point helps in calming the nervous system.
6. Chin (CH): Midway between the bottom of the lower lip and the chin. It's effective for feelings of confusion and uncertainty.
7. Beginning of the Collarbone (CB): Just below the hard ridge of your collarbone. Tapping here provides relief from emotional blockages.
8. Under the Arm (UA): Located about four inches beneath the armpit. Useful for self-esteem and fear issues.
9. Wrist Point (WR): The point where you would take your pulse on the wrist. It helps in managing stress and emotional distress.

The Setup Statement

Crafting an effective setup statement is foundational in EFT. This statement should acknowledge the problem and also include a phrase of self-acceptance, such as, "Even though I feel overwhelmed by this anxiety, I deeply and completely accept myself." This affirmation is crucial as it helps to maintain a balance between acknowledging the issue and fostering an attitude of self-compassion and acceptance, which is essential for emotional healing.

Sequential Flow

Begin your tapping sequence by repeating your setup statement three times while continuously tapping on the Karate Chop point on the side of your hand. This helps to prime your energy system for the session. Proceed by tapping about five to seven times on each point in the above sequence, starting from the top of the head and moving down to the wrist. While tapping, repeat a reminder phrase related to your setup statement, such as "this anxiety" or "my worry." This will help keep your focus on the issue at hand.

After you have tapped each point, take a deep breath and reassess the intensity of your problem. Rate your emotional or physical discomfort again on a scale from 0 to 10. Repeat the tapping sequence if necessary, adjusting your setup statement to reflect any change in your feelings or symptoms. This reassessment is crucial as it shows the shifts in your emotional or physical state, providing tangible proof of EFTs impact.

Visual Element: Diagram of Tapping Poin

Below is a detailed diagram of the tapping points to aid your learning and ensure accuracy in your tapping technique. This visual guide serves as a handy reference you can come back to at any time to refresh your memory of the location of each point, ensuring your tapping sessions are as effective as possible.

By understanding and practicing this primary tapping sequence, you equip yourself with a powerful tool to manage various emotional and physical challenges. This sequence is the foundation upon which other more specialized tapping routines are built, making it an essential skill for anyone beginning their EFT journey. As you become more comfortable with these techniques, you'll be able to handle previously daunting challenges with ease and confidence, tapping into your inner strength and resilience.

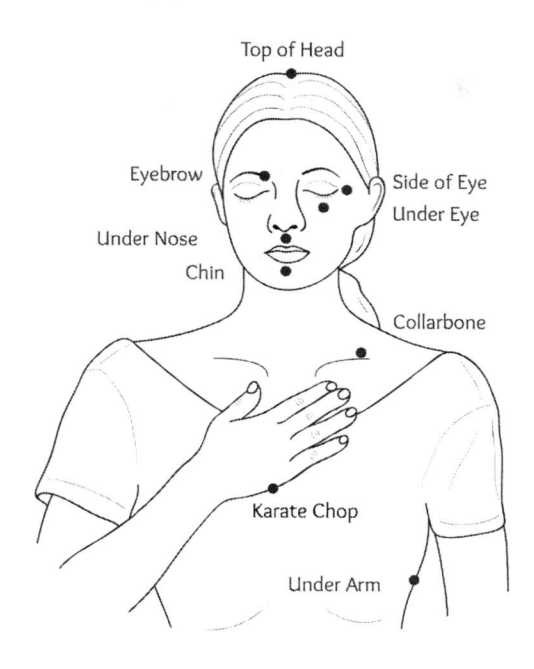

EFT Tapping Points

3.2 TAPPING FOR DAILY STRESS RELIEF: A ROUTINE TO UNWIND

In the fast-paced rhythm of modern life, stress can creep into your day with surprising ease, whether it's the morning rush, the endless emails, or the evening wind-down that doesn't quite go as planned. Integrating a simple, daily tapping routine for stress relief can profoundly alter how you experience and manage these daily pressures. Ideally, this routine should be performed twice a day—once in the morning to prepare your mind and body for the day's challenges and once in the evening to release accumulated stress and ensure a restful sleep. Each session need not be lengthy; even a few minutes can be sufficient to reset your emotional state.

To tailor this routine to your specific needs, identify the parts of your day that consistently provoke stress. Is it during your commute, midday meetings, or late at night when you struggle to disconnect from the day's responsibilities? Once identified, create personalized setup statements that directly address these stressors. For instance, if you find morning preparations chaotic, your setup statement might be, "Even though I feel overwhelmed by my morning routine, I deeply and completely accept myself and choose to find peace." This personalization of the setup statement is crucial—it acknowledges your feelings and affirms your self-acceptance, directly targeting the emotional aspect of your stress.

Enhancing your stress relief tapping routine with relaxation techniques can significantly amplify its benefits. Incorporating deep breathing exercises into your tapping sessions is particularly effective. Begin each session by taking three deep breaths—inhale slowly through your nose, allowing your abdomen to expand fully, and exhale through your mouth, releasing all the air and some of your tension. Continue to breathe deeply as you tap through the points, focusing on the sensation of each breath and each tap. This combination helps to center your mind, making the tapping process more meditative and powerful.

Let's explore a practical example of how you might use tapping to manage a common daily stressor: managing work-related stress. Picture yourself during a typical workday, feeling the pressure of impending deadlines and a crowded inbox. Your setup statement could be, "Even though my workload stresses me, I deeply and completely accept myself and choose to feel calm and focused." As you tap on each point, visualize your stress diminishing with each tap and breath, envisioning your day flowing more smoothly. This visualization technique not only helps to deepen the relaxation effect but also engages your brain's ability to manifest the calm and focus you desire.

Adopting this routine and adapting it to fit the specific rhythms and challenges of your day will equip you with a powerful tool that manages stress and enhances your overall well-being. This daily practice of tapping, personalized to your life's specifics and enhanced with techniques that deepen its impact, becomes a cornerstone of stress management and a balanced, emotionally healthy way of life. As you become more adept at identifying stressors and crafting effective setup statements, you'll find that what once seemed like overwhelming obstacles become manageable, tackled with calmness and resilience developed through your dedicated tapping practice.

3.3 QUICK TAPPING SOLUTIONS FOR SUDDEN ANXIETY

Anxiety often strikes without warning, transforming an otherwise ordinary moment into one of overwhelming stress. Recognizing what triggers these sudden bouts of anxiety is crucial in managing them effectively. Triggers can vary widely, including a looming deadline, an unexpected phone call, or even a particular social setting. The key to utilizing EFT tapping for sudden anxiety effectively is first to pinpoint these triggers. Reflect on recent instances when you felt a wave of anxiety. What were you doing? Who were you with? What thoughts were racing through your mind? Identifying patterns in these answers can help you anticipate and prepare for potential anxiety triggers.

Once triggers are identified, the goal is to manage anxiety swiftly and discreetly using a condensed version of the EFT tapping routine. This rapid response is crucial in preventing anxiety from escalating. Start by focusing on four main tapping points that are most accessible and can be tapped discreetly: the top of the head, the side of the hand (karate chop point), under the eye, and under the arm. This shortened routine allows for quick intervention that can be performed almost anywhere, from a busy office to a public transport system.

You should develop a set of portable, potent reminder phrases for each selected tapping point. These phrases should be short, specific, and easy to remember. Phrases like "calm and control" or "release this anxiety" can be effective. The simplicity and focus of these phrases help maintain your concentration on the tapping and breathing rather than the anxiety itself, facilitating a quicker return to calm. Practice these phrases as part of your regular tapping routine so that they come to mind quickly when you're under stress.

Now, let's consider how to apply these techniques in real-life situations where sudden anxiety might strike. Picture yourself about to give a presentation when suddenly, anxiety hits. Excuse yourself briefly, find a quiet corner, and perform your rapid tapping routine using the shortened sequence and prepared phrases. If you're in a situation where leaving isn't possible, such as during a stressful commute on public transport, use the karate chop point — a less noticeable tapping point — and focus on your breathing. Visualize each breath flowing to the point under your hand, carrying calmness with each tap. This method not only helps in managing the immediate symptoms of anxiety but also empowers you to regain control over your emotional state, no matter where you are or what situation you find yourself in.

By mastering these quick tapping solutions, you equip yourself with a powerful tool that brings considerable relief during unexpected moments of anxiety. This approach minimizes the disruption caused by such episodes and enhances your confidence and ability to handle stress, knowing you have the tools to regain balance at your fingertips. As you continue to practice these techniques, you'll find that your response to sudden anxiety becomes more automatic and effective, allowing you to maintain your composure and presence of mind even under pressure.

3.4 INTEGRATING AFFIRMATIONS WITH YOUR TAPPING PRACTICE

Integrating affirmations into your Emotional Freedom Techniques (EFT) sessions can significantly enhance the transformative power of tapping. Affirmations are positive, empowering statements that, when spoken with conviction, can help to shift your mindset and reinforce positive thinking. This psychological shift is crucial because it supports reprogramming your subconscious mind, fostering a landscape where positive changes can take root and flourish. By affirming your worth, capabilities, or calmness, you instruct your mind to adopt these attitudes, which can dramatically alter how you perceive and react to the world around you.

Creating effective affirmations is both a science and an art. To craft affirmations that resonate deeply with your personal aspirations or challenges, identify the negative beliefs or emotions you often encounter. These might be thoughts like "I am not good enough" or "I can't handle this stress." Transform these into positive, present-tense statements that promote acceptance and growth. For example, "I am enough just as I am" or "I handle stress gracefully and easily." The key here is to ensure that your affirmations are positive, framed in the present tense, and precise. This clarity and positivity help to counteract the negativity that can often cloud your subconscious directly.

Incorporating these affirmations into your tapping routine involves a mindful approach where each affirmation is focused on while tapping each point. Begin by selecting an affirmation that feels particularly potent for the issue. As you start your tapping sequence at the top of the head, gently recite your affirmation, allowing the words to sync with each tap. This method ensures that as you tap on each point, the vibrational energy of the affirmation is being embedded in your subconscious, enhancing the emotional resonance and deepening the impact of the session. For instance, while tapping under the eye, an area often associated with emotional pain, repeating an affirmation like "I release emotional pain with ease" can be particularly powerful.

Let's explore sample affirmations tailored to common issues such as self-esteem, anxiety, and achieving personal goals to give you a clearer picture of how this can be integrated into a routine. For self-esteem, an affirmation such as "I am worthy of love and respect" can be transformative. When tapping on the underarm, a point linked with self-esteem and self-acceptance, repeat this affirmation to reinforce feelings of self-worth. For anxiety, use an affirmation like "I am calm and at peace" while tapping on the collarbone, an area that helps soothe the nervous system. Lastly, for goal achievement, affirmations like "I am capable and successful in achieving my goals" can be repeated while tapping on the top of the head to instill a strong sense of capability and potential.

These examples illustrate how affirmations can be woven into the fabric of your tapping routines, each enhancing the other's effectiveness. This integration amplifies the benefits received from each session and makes the practice a deeply custom and personally enriching experience. As you become more accustomed to using affirmations within your tapping practice, you may find that they begin to naturally integrate into your everyday thought patterns, gradually replacing the negative self-talk that can often hinder personal growth and well-being.

In conclusion, this exploration of affirmations within the framework of EFT highlights a powerful tool for personal transformation. By understanding and utilizing the principles of positive affirmations in conjunction with the tapping points, you equip yourself with a dual force capable of challenging and changing the deep-seated beliefs that shape your reality. As you progress in your practice, these techniques will likely become integral to your emotional freedom and personal fulfillment journey. The next chapter will build on these foundational skills, guiding you through addressing specific emotional challenges with EFT and enhancing your ability to navigate life's ups and downs with resilience and grace.

CHAPTER 4

ADDRESSING EMOTIONAL CHALLENGES WITH EFT

Imagine you are standing at the edge of a serene lake, its surface smooth and undisturbed. Now, envision throwing a small stone into the center of this calm water. Watch as the ripples slowly expand outward, reaching further and further from the point of impact. This image mirrors the effect anxiety can have on our lives: a single worry or fear, seemingly small and manageable, can send waves through our entire being, affecting our peace of mind, physical health, and even our interactions with others. Emotional Freedom Techniques (EFT) offers a way to smooth these ripples back into calmness. This chapter focuses on one of the most common emotional challenges: anxiety. Here, you'll learn how to identify your anxiety triggers, create effective tapping scripts, and employ progressive tapping techniques to regain your tranquility.

4.1 TAPPING AWAY ANXIETY: SPECIFIC TECHNIQUES AND SCRIPTS

Identifying Anxiety Triggers

The first step in using EFT to manage anxiety effectively is to identify your specific triggers. These triggers can vary widely—they might be situations, thoughts, or sensory inputs that spark anxiety. To identify yours, start by recalling recent instances when you felt anxious. What was happening around you? Who were you with? What thoughts were going through your mind? It's crucial to note not only the psychological triggers but also the physical sensations associated with your anxiety. Do you feel a tightness in your chest or perhaps a knot in your stomach? Recognizing these signs will help you to address both the mental and physical aspects of your anxiety during your EFT sessions.

Script Creation for Anxiety

Once you've identified your triggers and associated sensations, the next step is to create personalized tapping scripts. These scripts should be specific to your experiences and feelings. Begin with a setup statement acknowledging your anxiety and affirming your acceptance of yourself, such as, "Even though I feel anxious when I think about my upcoming exam, I deeply and completely accept myself." Follow this by crafting reminder phrases you will repeat at each tapping point, like "this exam anxiety" or "the stress about my exam." These phrases help maintain your focus on the issue during the tapping process.

Progressive Tapping Technique

For a more nuanced approach to anxiety, you can use a progressive tapping technique. This method involves starting with a general tapping script that addresses your anxiety and then gradually moving to more specific issues. For instance, begin with a setup statement that targets your general feeling of anxiety, and as you tap through the points, gradually shift your focus to the more specific anxiety about an upcoming social event or a work presentation. This technique allows for a layered approach to emotional relief, starting from broad concerns and moving towards particular anxieties, facilitating a thorough and effective resolution.

Reinforcement through Repetition

The key to lasting change with EFT is consistency. Regular practice of your anxiety-specific tapping routines helps condition your mind and body to respond to stress with calmness and clarity. Make it a habit to tap daily, especially when you feel less anxious. This preventive practice helps build your emotional resilience, making you better equipped to handle stressors as they arise. Over time, this consistent repetition deepens the pathways of calm and control in your brain, making them the default routes your mind takes in stressful situations.

Interactive Element: Journaling Your Progress

To enhance your understanding and track the effectiveness of your tapping, maintain a journal dedicated to your EFT sessions. After each tapping sequence, write down the intensity of your anxiety before and after tapping, note any changes in your physical sensations, and reflect on how your responses to anxiety triggers may be evolving. This record not only provides you with insight into your progress but also reinforces your commitment to managing your anxiety through EFT. Reviewing your journal over time, you likely notice patterns and improvements that can further refine your tapping practices.

Through these tailored techniques and consistent practice, EFT equips you with the tools to smooth out the ripples of anxiety, restoring peace and balance to your mental and physical state. As you progress in your practice, remember the image of the lake—calm, serene, and undisturbed. With each tapping session, you are working towards reclaiming this tranquility in your own life, mastering the art of self-regulation and emotional resilience.

4.2 OVERCOMING FEAR AND PHOBIAS WITH TARGETED TAPPING

Fear can be as simple as a slight nervousness or as complex as a paralyzing phobia. Regardless of its scale, fear profoundly affects how you live and enjoy life. Tapping, or Emotional Freedom Techniques (EFT), provides a powerful method to confront these fears directly, allowing you to gradually regain control over your emotions and actions. The first crucial step in using EFT to tackle your fears is clearly mapping them out. Start by identifying what exactly it is that scares you. Is it heights, public speaking, certain animals, or a specific situation like driving or flying? Understanding the root of your fear or phobia and recognizing the triggers that spark this fear is essential. Triggers could be anything—a sound, a place, an action, or even a time of day. Once you've pinpointed these elements, you're better prepared to structure your tapping sessions effectively.

After identifying what you are afraid of, the next step in the EFT process focuses on tapping points that are particularly effective in mitigating fear responses. Two primary meridian points that help address fear are the top of the head (TOH) and under the nose (UN). Tapping on the TOH point can broadly influence your body's energy system, impacting psychological and emotional aspects, and is especially useful for general fear. The UN point, located between the upper lip and the nose, is typically associated with fostering emotional calmness and is particularly effective in reducing anxiety driven by fears. When you tap on these points, you stimulate meridian pathways that can help calm the amygdala, the part of your brain that plays a crucial role in processing emotions related to fear and anxiety.

Integrating visualization techniques with tapping enhances the effectiveness of your sessions. For instance, if you fear public speaking, you might visualize yourself standing on a stage, feeling calm, and speaking confidently. As you hold this image in your mind, begin your tapping sequence. This visualization reinforces your desired positive outcome and aligns your subconscious mind with your conscious efforts. By visualizing success, you're programming your mind to act in accordance with this new script, diminishing the instinctual fear response and replacing it with a new, positive association.

Using incremental exposure scripts in your tapping routine can effectively solidify your progress in overcoming fears. This method involves gradually exposing yourself to your fear within the safe environment of your mind combined with the tapping process. Start with less intimidating aspects of your fear and slowly build up to more challenging aspects. For example, if you are afraid of flying, initially visualize yourself preparing for a flight, then being at the airport, boarding the plane, and finally, taking off. Each stage should be tackled separately in different tapping sessions. This gradual exposure helps desensitize your fear response over time, making the experience less daunting when you finally face it.

By mapping your fears, utilizing specific tapping points, combining tapping with visualization, and employing incremental exposure scripts, you equip yourself with a robust strategy to confront and conquer your fears. This proactive approach not only diminishes the immediate anxiety associated with specific phobias but also builds a foundation of courage and self-assurance that enhances your overall quality of life. As you continue to apply these techniques, each step forward in this tapping journey significantly dismantles the barriers fear has built around your life, opening up new avenues for personal freedom and fulfillment.

4.3 EFT FOR MANAGING DEPRESSION: A GENTLE APPROACH

Depression can often be like a shadow, subtly influencing your thoughts and actions without a clear, visible presence. Recognizing the emotional and physical symptoms of depression is the first critical step in managing it effectively through Emotional Freedom Techniques (EFT). These symptoms can range widely from persistent sadness and feelings of emptiness to physical manifestations such as fatigue, changes in appetite, or sleep disturbances. Some might experience irritability or an inability to find pleasure in activities once enjoyed, while others might find themselves wrestling with feelings of worthlessness or disproportionate guilt. Understanding that these varied symptoms are interconnected facets of depression is fundamental. By acknowledging these signs, you set the groundwork for a targeted EFT approach that addresses both the emotional and physical aspects of depression, paving the way for more comprehensive healing.

One compelling application of EFT in managing depression revolves around fostering self-compassion. For many experiencing depression, a harsh inner critic can amplify feelings of low self-worth and inadequacy. Developing a tapping routine centered on self-compassion involves crafting setup statements that directly counteract this critical inner voice. For instance, a statement like, "Even though I feel unworthy, I deeply and completely accept myself and recognize my value," can be profoundly transformative. As you tap through the points, reinforce this affirmation, allowing each tap to resonate as a confirmation of your inherent worth. This practice not only helps to alleviate depressive symptoms but also nurtures an inner environment where kindness and self-acceptance can flourish. Over time, these positive affirmations become ingrained, gradually replacing the negative self-perceptions that often accompany depression.

Incorporating daily tapping rituals is another effective strategy for managing depression. These rituals act as both preventative and responsive measures. On days when you might feel the weight of depression more acutely, having a specific tapping routine can provide immediate relief. Create a set of tapping routines that address various aspects of your depression. For example, one routine might focus on alleviating sadness, while another might aim to restore energy levels when you're feeling particularly fatigued. Start your day with a tapping session that prepares you for the day's challenges, emphasizing resilience and energy. Before bedtime, another routine can focus on releasing the day's stresses, ensuring a restful sleep. By integrating these rituals into your daily schedule, you create consistent touchpoints for emotional maintenance, which can help stabilize mood fluctuations and prevent the deep lows that often accompany depression.

Linking thoughts to physical sensations is a unique aspect of EFT that is particularly beneficial in treating depression. The mind-body connection is powerful, and physical sensations often accompany emotional pain. For instance, anxiety might manifest as a tightening in the chest, or sadness might feel like a heaviness in the shoulders.

Focus on these physical sensations in your tapping sessions as you address the emotional thoughts. Begin with a setup statement that acknowledges both the physical sensation and the emotional pain, such as, "Even though my chest feels tight with anxiety, and I feel overwhelmed, I deeply and completely accept myself and choose to feel calm and relaxed." As you tap each point, imagine the physical tension dissolving, and visualize your body releasing the emotional and physical pain. This dual focus not only provides relief but also reinforces the understanding of how closely your emotions and physical body are linked, promoting a holistic approach to managing depression.

By carefully recognizing the signs of depression, fostering self-compassion, integrating daily tapping rituals, and linking emotional thoughts to physical sensations, EFT offers a gentle yet powerful approach to managing depression. This method provides temporary relief and a path toward long-term wellness, empowering you to take control of your emotional health in a compassionate and self-affirming way. Through regular practice, these techniques build a foundation of emotional resilience, enabling you to face life's crazy twists with a renewed sense of strength and balance.

4.4 HEALING EMOTIONAL TRAUMA THROUGH EFT

When addressing emotional trauma with Emotional Freedom Techniques (EFT), it is crucial to approach each session with a trauma-informed lens. This approach is foundational in ensuring that the tapping process aids the healing journey without inadvertently causing re-traumatization. Trauma-informed EFT acknowledges the complexity and sensitivity of trauma, recognizing that traditional tapping sequences, while beneficial for many emotional issues, need to be adapted to meet the unique needs of individuals who have experienced trauma. The essence of this approach is to tread gently, ensuring that each step in the tapping process is conducted with an awareness of its potential impact. This involves being attuned to how trauma can affect individuals differently, making it essential to tailor EFT sessions to each person's specific experiences and reactions.

Creating a safe space is the first critical step in trauma-focused EFT. This space is not just physical but also emotional. Physically, a quiet, private setting where you won't be disturbed is ideal. Emotionally, the space should feel secure and supportive, where vulnerability can be expressed without fear of judgment or harm. For many, the presence of a trusted therapist or a support system can provide the necessary feeling of safety required to explore deeply rooted traumas. If you're working through trauma alone, consider making your environment as comforting as possible—soft lighting, soothing music, or familiar objects can help create a sense of security.

The process of tapping for traumatic memories requires careful consideration and should always prioritize your comfort and emotional safety. Start by identifying a memory that feels significant but not overwhelmingly distressing. The goal is not to dive into the most painful memories first but to gradually work your way through less triggering experiences, building resilience as you go. Develop a tapping script for each memory that acknowledges the pain and affirms your strength and resilience. For instance, a script might start with, "Even though this memory is painful and hard to revisit, I deeply and completely accept myself and recognize my strength to heal." As you tap through the points, focus on maintaining a slow and gentle rhythm, allowing yourself to process the emotions that arise without rushing or forcing anything. It's important to pace the session according to your reactions—some days might allow for deeper exploration, while others might require a more gentle approach.

Integrating professional support with EFT is highly recommended, especially for deep-seated trauma. Professionals trained in trauma-informed care can provide the guidance and support necessary to navigate the complexities of trauma safely. They can help tailor EFT scripts to address specific traumatic experiences and offer support through difficult emotions that may arise during tapping. Additionally, they can integrate EFT with other therapeutic approaches to provide comprehensive care. Discuss how you can incorporate EFT into your sessions if you're already working with a therapist. For those new to therapy, seeking out a therapist who is familiar with EFT and understands the nuances of trauma therapy can be incredibly beneficial.

Textual Element: Checklist for Trauma-Informed Tapping

1. Ensure a Safe Environment: Confirm that the physical and emotional environment feels secure and supportive.
2. Begin with Less Intense Memories: Select traumatic memories that are not overwhelmingly distressing to start with.
3. Develop Gentle Tapping Scripts: Create scripts that acknowledge the trauma and reinforce your capacity for healing.
4. Pace According to Comfort: Listen to your emotional responses, adjusting the tapping pace to avoid overwhelming yourself.
5. Seek Professional Guidance: Consider working with a trauma-informed therapist to explore more profound traumatic memories safely.

By adhering to a trauma-informed approach, creating a safe tapping environment, carefully crafting scripts, and possibly integrating professional support, EFT becomes a powerful tool in the healing process from trauma. This careful, mindful approach ensures that tapping is a supportive, healing practice that respects trauma's profound impact on one's life.

Navigating through the chapters, we've explored various facets of using EFT to manage and heal from emotional challenges like anxiety, fears, depression, and trauma. Each section has provided specific techniques tailored to these issues, emphasizing the importance of customization and sensitivity to individual experiences. The subsequent chapters will build upon these foundations as we progress, exploring how EFT can enhance emotional freedom and well-being in everyday life. This journey through EFT is not just about overcoming challenges—it's about embracing a tool that fosters resilience, empowerment, and profound personal growth.

CHAPTER 5
TAPPING FOR PHYSICAL HEALTH

Imagine your body as a complex network of roads and highways. Now, picture traffic flow being disrupted due to roadblocks, leading to congestion and delays that affect the entire system. Similarly, chronic pain can be seen as a disruption in your body's natural flow of energy, causing discomfort and distress that can significantly impact your quality of life. Emotional Freedom Techniques (EFT), or tapping, offers a dynamic approach to navigating and clearing these blockages, restoring ease and flow within your body. This chapter delves into the intricate relationship between emotional stress and physical pain, guiding you through specific tapping techniques designed to alleviate chronic pain and enhance your overall well-being.

5.1 USING EFT TO ALLEVIATE CHRONIC PAIN

Understanding Pain and Emotions

Chronic pain often serves as more than just a physical symptom; it can also be a manifestation of unresolved emotional stress. The body and mind are intricately linked, and emotions like anxiety, sadness, or unresolved trauma can manifest physically as persistent pain. This phenomenon is rooted in the body's stress response, which, when continuously activated, can lead to inflammation and muscle tension, exacerbating pain conditions. EFT taps into this mind-body connection by addressing the emotional contributors to pain, easing the physical symptoms, and promoting emotional healing. As you tap on specific meridian points, you effectively send calming signals to the brain, reducing stress hormones like cortisol, and interrupting the pain cycle.

Specific Tapping Points for Pain Relief

Specific EFT tapping points have proven particularly beneficial in effectively targeting chronic pain. Two key points to focus on include the top of the head (TOH) and the beginning of the collarbone (CB). Tapping on the TOH point influences the entire body's energy system, making it an ideal starting point for addressing widespread pain or discomfort. The CB point, located just below where your collarbone meets your sternum, is crucial for alleviating stress and tension, common contributors to chronic pain. Here's how you can activate these points:

1. Top of the Head (TOH): Using the fingertips of one or both hands, gently tap around the crown of your head. This area is linked to general body balance and emotional release.

2. Beginning of the Collarbone (CB): Place your fingertips on the fleshy part below your collarbone and gently tap. This point is particularly effective for releasing deep-seated emotional stress and physical tension.

Regularly tapping these points encourages the release of pain and tension, fostering a sense of physical relief and emotional calm.

Creating Personalized Pain Relief Scripts

Personalizing your EFT scripts allows you to address the specific emotional aspects of your pain, enhancing the effectiveness of each tapping session. Begin by identifying the emotions tied to your pain—stress, anger, or sadness. Craft your setup statement to acknowledge these feelings and affirm your commitment to healing. For example, "Even though I feel overwhelmed by this back pain, I deeply and completely accept myself and am open to healing." As you tap through the points, repeat a reminder phrase that keeps you focused on releasing these emotions, such as "releasing the pain" or "letting go of the stress."

Case Studies and Success Stories

To illustrate the potential effectiveness of these techniques, consider the experience of Michael, a long-time sufferer of chronic back pain. After years of various treatments with limited success, Michael tried EFT as a last resort. He began tapping daily, focusing on releasing the anger and frustration associated with his pain. Within weeks, not only did his pain levels decrease significantly, but his general well-being improved as well. Stories like Michael's underscore the transformative potential of EFT in managing chronic pain, providing hope and a possible pathway to those seeking relief.

Textual Element: Reflection Section

Take a moment to reflect on any physical discomfort you currently experience and the emotions that might be contributing to it. How does your body feel when you are stressed or upset? Recognizing these connections can be the first step toward effective pain management with EFT. This self-awareness is a powerful tool, equipping you with the knowledge to tailor your tapping practice to your specific needs, fostering more profound healing and recovery.

5.2 EFT TECHNIQUES FOR HEADACHE RELIEF

Headaches, whether occasional or chronic, can disrupt your daily activities and significantly affect your quality of life. Understanding what triggers your headaches is an essential first step toward managing them effectively with Emotional Freedom Techniques (EFT). Common triggers include emotional stress, certain food items, environmental factors like bright lights or loud noises, and even posture-related issues. By identifying these triggers, you can more accurately target your EFT sessions to address the root causes of your headaches rather than just the symptoms. Start by keeping a headache diary where you note when each headache occurs, its intensity, what you ate, how you felt emotionally, and what you did. This record can help you spot patterns and pinpoint specific triggers. For instance, you might notice that your headaches tend to flare up after long periods at the computer, suggesting a link to posture and eye strain, or following stressful meetings, indicating a potential stress trigger.

Once you've identified potential triggers, you can apply EFT as an immediate relief measure during a headache. The goal is to focus on meridian points that reduce tension and promote relaxation. A simple yet effective tapping sequence for headache relief might begin at the top of the head, move to the eyebrow points, and then to the temples—areas often associated with tension headaches. Follow these steps for a quick relief routine:

1. Top of the Head: Start by tapping gently at the crown of your head. This point can help alleviate overall stress and reduce the feeling of pressure often associated with headaches.
2. Eyebrow Points: Move to the points at the start of your eyebrows, right above the nose. Tap here to release tension that accumulates in the forehead.
3. Temples: Gently tap around the temple area. This can be particularly soothing for headaches as it helps relax the muscles around the sides of your head.
4. Collarbone Points: Finish by tapping just under the collarbone. This area effectively calms the nervous system and can help diminish the intensity of headaches.

Incorporating these points into a regular tapping routine addresses the immediate discomfort and is a preventative strategy. Regular tapping can help manage stress levels—one of the most common triggers for headaches—thereby reducing the frequency and severity of headaches over time. Consider setting aside specific times each day for a brief tapping session, focusing on relaxation and stress management. Morning sessions can set a calm tone for the day, potentially warding off stress-induced headaches. In contrast, evening sessions can help release the day's tensions, ensuring better sleep and fewer morning headaches.

In addition to EFT, integrating specific lifestyle changes can enhance your ability to manage headaches. Hydration is critical in preventing headaches, as dehydration is a common trigger. Make sure to drink adequate amounts of water throughout the day. Similarly, adjusting your posture, especially if you spend long hours at a desk, can significantly impact you. Simple changes like adjusting the height of your monitor, using an ergonomic chair, or taking regular breaks to stretch can prevent the tension buildup that often leads to headaches. While seemingly small, these adjustments can dramatically improve your overall well-being and reduce reliance on pain medications or other interventions.

By taking a holistic approach to managing headaches through EFT, identifying triggers, applying targeted tapping techniques, maintaining a preventative routine, and making thoughtful lifestyle adjustments, you equip yourself with a comprehensive toolkit for managing this common yet disruptive ailment. This proactive and empowered approach alleviates physical discomfort and enhances your overall quality of life, ensuring that headaches no longer hold you back from enjoying your daily activities.

5.3 TAPPING TO ENHANCE ENERGY LEVELS

Feeling drained or lethargic can often signal that your body and emotional landscape need attention. Emotional blockages, such as unresolved anger, sadness, or anxiety, can significantly deplete your energy levels. These emotions can disrupt your body's energy system, much like a dam blocks a river's flow. When your emotional energy is blocked, it prevents your physical body from functioning optimally, leading to fatigue and decreased vitality. Emotional Freedom Techniques (EFT), or tapping, offers a method to clear these blockages, helping to restore your energy flow and rejuvenate your spirit.

One of the most effective ways to release these emotional blockages and boost your energy is by tapping on specific points known for their energizing properties. Two such points are the kidney meridian points on the lower back, just below the rib cage, and the sacral points near the base of the spine. These areas are particularly significant in traditional Chinese medicine because of their role in the vital energy and life force known as Qi. Activating these points through tapping can help stimulate energy flow throughout the body, enhancing overall vitality. To effectively activate these points, gently tap your fingertips and focus on breathing deeply. As you tap, visualize the energy flowing smoothly through these areas, washing away blockages and revitalizing your body.

To make the most of these benefits, incorporating a daily energy-boosting routine can be incredibly effective. Begin by setting aside a few minutes each morning to engage in a tapping session focused on clearing any emotional residue from the previous day and setting a positive tone for the day ahead. Start with the kidney and sacral points to activate your body's energy centers. Then, move to the chest and underarm points to open up the heart and lungs, which helps to invigorate your entire system. Incorporate affirmations reinforcing your intention to feel energized and alert, such as "I feel vibrant and full of energy." This routine not only helps to wake up your body but also clears your mind, making you more prepared to face the day's challenges.

The transformative power of EFT in boosting energy levels is not just anecdotal; it is supported by numerous success stories from individuals who have incorporated tapping into their daily routines. For instance, consider the experience of Linda, a freelance graphic designer who was constantly tired and struggling to meet deadlines. After beginning a daily tapping routine focused on the kidney and sacral points, Linda noticed a significant improvement in her energy levels within just a few weeks. She reported feeling more awake in the mornings and more productive throughout the day. Her story is just one of many that highlight how tapping can alleviate physical fatigue and bring a renewed sense of vitality and enthusiasm for life.

Understanding the connection between your emotions and energy levels and utilizing specific tapping points and routines can significantly enhance your vitality. This practice improves your physical energy and contributes to a more balanced and harmonious emotional state, allowing you to enjoy a more active and fulfilling life. As you continue to explore and apply these techniques, you may feel more energetic and emotionally resilient, ready to tackle whatever challenges come your way.

5.4 EFT FOR DIGESTIVE HEALTH: A HOLISTIC APPROACH

The intricate dance between our emotional well-being and our digestive health continues to fascinate and challenge both medical professionals and those of us keen on maintaining our health. It's often said that the gut is our second brain, and this isn't just a poetic metaphor. The gut-brain connection is a scientifically recognized pathway through which emotional stress can significantly impact digestive functioning. When stressed, your body's fight or flight response is activated, diverting energy from the digestive system and leading to disruptions like bloating, indigestion, or other gastrointestinal discomforts. This is where Emotional Freedom Techniques (EFT), or tapping, comes into play, offering a method to ease both the psychological and physiological symptoms intertwined with digestive issues.

Embarking on a tapping routine specifically designed for digestive relief can be transformative. The key points to focus on include the abdomen, which directly correlates with digestive health, and the collarbone point, which helps reduce overall stress levels—a significant trigger for digestive complaints. Here's a simple routine to follow:

1. Start with the Collarbone (CB) Point: Tap gently just beneath the collarbone. This helps to calm the stress response, which is often a precursor to digestive discomfort.
2. Move to the Abdomen Points: Place your hands gently on your abdomen and tap lightly. Focus on areas that feel particularly tense or uncomfortable.
3. Under the Rib (UR) Points: Located just below the ribs, these points are crucial for addressing upper digestive tract issues like heartburn or reflux.
4. End at the Lower Abdomen Points: These are situated around the belly button and lower. They are key in addressing issues in the lower digestive tract.

While tapping, focus on deep, rhythmic breathing and use affirmations that reinforce a message of calm and healing, such as "I release stress from my body, and my stomach is calm." This combination of tapping and affirmations helps to regulate the nervous system, reducing the stress that exacerbates digestive issues and promoting a more harmonious gut function.

Incorporating dietary considerations into your routine enhances the effectiveness of EFT in managing digestive health. A balanced diet with adequate fiber, probiotics, and hydration naturally supports digestive health. However, each person's body is unique, and certain foods might trigger discomfort. Here, tapping can again assist you in maintaining a more mindful relationship with food. Use tapping to explore and possibly eliminate emotional eating habits or to curb cravings that lead to discomfort. An affirmation like "I choose foods that nourish and comfort my body" can be powerful. Additionally, consider keeping a food diary alongside your tapping sessions to identify correlations between your eating, your emotions, and how your body reacts. Combining tapping with dietary mindfulness, this holistic approach provides a comprehensive strategy for maintaining optimal digestive health.

Chronic digestive conditions such as Irritable Bowel Syndrome (IBS) can benefit from integrating EFT into the management plan. For chronic conditions, consistency with tapping is critical. Regular tapping can help manage the stress that often triggers or worsens symptoms associated with conditions like IBS. In these cases, tapping should be seen as a complementary therapy alongside medical treatment prescribed by healthcare professionals. It's important to communicate with your healthcare provider about using EFT as part of your treatment plan, ensuring it fits seamlessly with other interventions.

In this exploration of EFT for digestive health, we've seen how tapping can address the complex interplay of stress, emotion, and physical symptoms that characterize digestive issues. You can significantly enhance your digestive health by using targeted tapping routines, integrating mindful eating, and applying EFT as a complementary therapy for chronic conditions. This holistic approach alleviates physical symptoms and promotes a deeper, more harmonious connection between your mind and body, improving overall health and well-being.

As this chapter concludes, the journey through EFT applications in enhancing physical health reveals the profound impact this technique can have on your body and overall quality of life. By addressing the root emotional causes of physical symptoms, EFT offers a pathway to more profound healing and enduring health. The next chapter will explore how EFT can be adapted for special populations, ensuring that everyone, regardless of their specific challenges or conditions, can benefit from this versatile and powerful tool.

CHAPTER 6

ENHANCING SELF-CONFIDENCE AND PERSONAL GROWTH

Imagine stepping into a room full of mirrors, each reflecting an image of you. Now, imagine each mirror subtly distorts your reflection, some making you look taller, others wider, some dimming your smile, while others brighten your eyes. This room of mirrors can be linked to the various facets of self-esteem, each reflecting a slightly different version of who you are, filtered through the lens of your experiences, beliefs, and emotions. Emotional Freedom Techniques (EFT) or tapping offers you the tools to adjust these mirrors, aligning them to reflect a more accurate, empowered, and positive image of yourself. In this chapter, we delve into the intricate process of building self-esteem through EFT, highlighting methods to identify and remove the distortions that cloud your self-perception, thereby enhancing your confidence and facilitating personal growth.

6.1 BUILDING SELF-ESTEEM: TAPPING INTO YOUR POTENTIAL

Identifying Self-Esteem Blockers

The journey towards bolstering self-esteem begins with identifying the barriers that hold you back, often rooted in negative self-beliefs. These beliefs might manifest as recurring thoughts like "I am not good enough," "I don't deserve happiness," or "I can't succeed." Such thoughts are potent, self-fulfilling prophecies that not only skew your self-image but also limit your potential. To unearth these deep-seated beliefs, reflect on situations where you feel particularly vulnerable or inadequate. Notice the narratives that play in your mind during these moments. Journaling these thoughts can be incredibly revealing and serves as the first step in your tapping journey. By articulating these negative beliefs, you set the stage for targeted EFT sessions that directly address and dismantle these destructive narratives.

Tapping Scripts for Self-Acceptance

Once you have identified your self-esteem blockers, the next step involves creating tapping scripts that foster acceptance and counteract negative self-talk. A basic script might start with you acknowledging the negative belief while integrating a positive affirmation: "Even though I believe I am not worthy of love, I deeply and completely accept myself and recognize my inherent worth." Repeat this affirmation as you tap through the points from the top of the head down to the collarbone, allowing the words to resonate with each tap. The physical stimulation of EFT points, combined with vocal affirmations, helps rewire emotional responses and gradually erodes the foundation of your self-limiting beliefs.

Affirmations for Self-Esteem

Affirmations are powerful tools in reinforcing the positive changes initiated by tapping. These should be positive, present-tense statements that reflect the qualities or achievements you aspire to embody, such as "I am capable and confident" or "I succeed in my endeavors." Integrate these affirmations into your tapping routine by repeating them aloud with conviction at each tapping point. The repetition of positive affirmations during tapping helps embed these empowering beliefs into your subconscious, gradually replacing the old, negative narratives that have hindered your self-esteem.

Reflective Practices Post-Tapping

To solidify the gains from your tapping sessions, engage in reflective practices such as journaling or meditative contemplation. After each tapping session, take a moment to write down any shifts in thoughts, feelings, or physical sensations you experienced. Reflect on how your perception of yourself might have changed, even subtly. This practice reinforces the positive impacts of tapping and encourages a habit of self-awareness and mindful reflection, crucial components in the ongoing journey of personal growth and self-improvement.

Textual Element: Self-Esteem Journaling Prompts

To enhance your reflective practice, here are some journaling prompts that can guide your exploration of self-esteem post-tapping:

1. What negative beliefs did I focus on today?
2. How do I feel about this belief after tapping?
3. What new, positive belief can replace the old one?
4. How can I reinforce this new belief in my daily life?

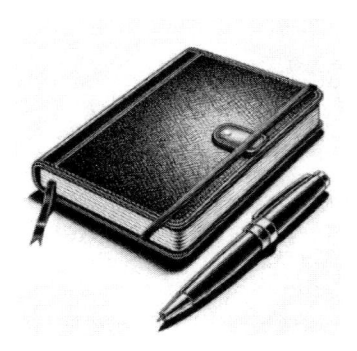

These prompts serve as tools for reflection and as beacons that guide your progress, illuminating the path from self-doubt to self-assurance. As you continue to use these tools, you'll find that what once seemed insurmountable barriers to your self-esteem become stepping stones to a more confident and empowered self.

By systematically addressing the components of building self-esteem through EFT, you equip yourself with the skills to reshape how you see yourself, enhancing your self-confidence and capacity to thrive and succeed in various aspects of your life. This transformative process is not just about changing how you feel in the moment; it's about cultivating a deeper, enduring sense of self-worth and potential that propels you forward on your journey of personal growth.

6.2 OVERCOMING IMPOSTER SYNDROME WITH EFT

Imposter syndrome is a common psychological phenomenon where individuals doubt their accomplishments and fear being exposed as a "fraud" despite evident success. This syndrome can manifest in various ways, from persistent self-doubt and perfectionism to the inability to realistically assess one's competence and skills. Those experiencing imposter syndrome attribute their success to external factors like luck, and they fear that others will eventually uncover them as lacking actual ability or qualifications. Understanding that these feelings are widespread can be the first step toward overcoming them. It's especially prevalent among high achievers and can significantly impact your professional and personal life, leading to stress, anxiety, and missed opportunities.

We target the specific feelings associated with this complex condition to address imposter syndrome with Emotional Freedom Techniques (EFT). One effective way to do this is through a tailored tapping sequence that addresses the core feelings of imposter syndrome, such as fear of being exposed or beliefs of not being good enough. Start this sequence by identifying the most pressing thought that fuels your imposter syndrome. For example, you might feel like you don't truly deserve your job or accolades despite your hard work and the praise you receive.

Begin your tapping session with a setup statement acknowledging this fear and integrating a positive affirmation. You might say, "Even though I don't truly deserve my role and fear others will find out, I deeply and completely accept myself and recognize my competence and worth." As you tap on each of the key EFT points —starting from the top of the head (TOH), moving through the eyebrow (EB), side of the eye (SE), under the eye (UE), under the nose (UN), the chin (CH), the beginning of the collarbone (CB), and under the arm (UA)—repeat a reminder phrase such as "this fear of being exposed" to maintain focus on this specific issue.

Incorporating role-playing scenarios into your tapping routine can further enhance the effectiveness of combating imposter syndrome. Visualize a specific situation where you might typically feel like an imposter. For instance, imagine you are about to lead a meeting or present a project. As you tap, envision yourself conducting these tasks with confidence and authority. Feel the success and acceptance from your peers and superiors. This visualization reinforces the positive outcomes of your actions and helps reprogram your subconscious to associate these situations with competence and success rather than fear and doubt.

Developing long-term strategies for resilience against imposter feelings is crucial for lasting change. Regular tapping can significantly alter ingrained belief systems that contribute to imposter syndrome. By consistently practicing the targeted tapping sequences and role-playing scenarios, you can gradually shift your self-perception from that of a "fraud" to an authentic achiever who recognizes and owns their successes. It's also beneficial to reflect on each tapping session to observe progress and areas that need further work. Maintaining a journal where you document these reflections and the evolving feelings about your abilities and achievements can be incredibly supportive.

Imposter Syndrome Tapping Checklist

To aid in your regular practice, here's a checklist to ensure each session is as effective as possible:

1. Identify the Triggering Situation: What specific event or thought brought on feelings of imposter syndrome?
2. Craft a Focused Setup Statement: Create a statement acknowledging the imposter feeling and integrating a self-acceptance affirmation.
3. Choose Specific Reminder Phrases: Pick phrases that resonate with your feelings of being an imposter to use while tapping through the points.
4. Engage in Role-Playing: Visualize a scenario where you successfully overcome your imposter syndrome.
5. Reflect and Journal Post-Tapping: Note any changes in

your feelings or perceptions about your abilities and accomplishments.

By methodically applying these strategies, EFT provides a robust framework for managing and overcoming the debilitating effects of imposter syndrome. This approach empowers you to reclaim your achievements as your own and to walk confidently in your professional and personal life, free from the shadows of doubt that imposter syndrome casts. As you continue to use these techniques, you'll likely find that the voice of self-doubt becomes quieter, and your authentic, deserving self emerges more clearly with each tapping session.

6.3 TAPPING FOR PUBLIC SPEAKING AND PERFORMANCE ANXIETY

Public speaking is a common source of stress and anxiety for many people, often triggering a range of fears from being judged harshly by an audience to forgetting one's lines during a crucial moment. Physical symptoms such as shaking, sweating, or a racing heart can also accompany this anxiety, making the experience even more daunting. Understanding and addressing these fears is the first step toward gaining confidence in your public speaking abilities. Begin by closely examining your past experiences with public speaking. Identify the moments that felt most uncomfortable or where anxiety seemed to peak. Was it right before stepping onto the stage or during a question-and-answer session? Pinpointing these moments helps tailor your tapping approach to be as effective as possible.

Once you've identified your specific fears, you can develop a focused tapping routine before any speaking engagement. This routine should be designed to reduce immediate anxiety and increase mental clarity and focus. Start by selecting a quiet place to spend a few minutes uninterrupted. Begin with the setup statement acknowledging your fear and asserting your commitment to calm and clarity. You might say something like, "Even though I feel nervous about speaking in front of my peers, I deeply and completely accept myself and choose to speak clearly and confidently." As you tap through the points, from the top of your head to under your arms, repeat a reminder phrase such as "calm and clear" to help maintain focus on your intention to remain composed and articulate.

Visualization techniques can significantly enhance the effects of tapping by engaging the imagination to reinforce positive outcomes. While tapping, visualize yourself standing before the audience, delivering your speech with confidence and poise. See yourself speaking clearly, making eye contact, and receiving nods of approval and smiles from the audience. Feel the satisfaction of a well-received presentation. This mental rehearsal primes your subconscious to act in accordance with this positive scenario, reducing anxiety and boosting self-confidence. The combination of tapping and visualization addresses the physical symptoms of stress and the mental barriers to effective public speaking, creating a powerful dual strategy to enhance your performance.

After your performance, it's beneficial to use tapping to process and release any residual stress and to integrate feedback constructively. This post-performance tapping can help you solidify the positive aspects of your experience and learn from any mistakes without harsh self-judgment. Begin by acknowledging how you feel after the speech, perhaps noting any moments of anxiety or particular successes. Tap through the points while focusing on

ENHANCING SELF-CONFIDENCE AND PERSONAL GROWTH

releasing negative emotions and reinforcing the positive aspects of your performance. For instance, if you stumbled over a part of your speech but recovered well, you might tap on the affirmation, "Even though I lost my place, I am proud of myself for recovering gracefully, and I learn and grow with every speaking opportunity."

Using EFT to manage public speaking and performance anxiety offers a practical and effective method to cope with the immediate symptoms of anxiety and build a foundation of confidence that improves overall performance. Through regular practice, both before and after performances, you can transform what was once a source of dread into an opportunity for personal growth and professional development. Each successful application of these techniques reinforces your ability to handle public speaking scenarios with increasing ease and effectiveness, contributing to a more confident and capable you.

6.4 USING EFT TO SET AND ACHIEVE PERSONAL GOALS

Setting and achieving goals is akin to planting a garden. It begins with envisioning what you wish to cultivate, preparing the soil, planting the seeds, and then consistently tending to your plants by watering them and removing any weeds that might impede their growth. Similarly, Emotional Freedom Techniques (EFT) can be used to nurture your goals from inception to fruition. It starts with clearly defining what you want to achieve, preparing your mental ground by clearing self-limiting beliefs, planting seeds of motivation, and consistently nurturing your progress with positive affirmations and tapping routines.

Clarifying and Setting Goals

The first step in any successful endeavor is to define your goals clearly. Specificity and measurability are critical components of effective goal-setting. For instance, rather than setting a vague goal like "I want to be successful," specify what success looks like to you. Is it a promotion at work, starting your own business, or writing a book? Once you have a specific goal in mind, ensure it is measurable. For example, if your goal is to write a book, you could set a quantifiable objective, such as writing a chapter each month.

Additionally, it's crucial to ensure that your goals align with your values. This alignment makes the goal more meaningful and increases your intrinsic motivation. Start by listing what truly matters to you and see how these can be woven into your goals. This practice clarifies what you want to achieve and why you want to achieve it, adding a layer of emotional motivation that can propel you forward.

Tapping to Overcome Obstacles

Every path to a goal usually comes with obstacles, be it procrastination, fear of failure, or a lack of motivation. EFT can be a powerful ally in overcoming these barriers. For instance, if procrastination is your hurdle, construct a tapping routine that addresses the root cause of your procrastination. A setup statement for this could be, "Even though I keep putting off starting my project, I deeply and completely accept myself and choose to feel motivated and focused." As you tap through the points, visualize yourself taking action and the positive outcomes of doing so. This visualization, coupled with tapping, helps reprogram your subconscious mind to align with your conscious goals, gradually reducing the urge to procrastinate.

Maintaining Focus and Motivation

Maintaining focus and motivation is crucial, especially when progress seems slow or obstacles seem insurmountable. EFT can be utilized to sustain your drive toward your goals. Create a tapping routine that reinforces your commitment and focus. Begin with a setup statement like, "Even though I feel like I'm not making progress, I deeply and completely accept myself and choose to remain focused and driven." Regularly tapping with this focus can help maintain your momentum, even during challenging times. This routine acts like a mental and emotional check-in that realigns your energies and reaffirms your commitment to your goals.

Celebrating Milestones with EFT

Recognizing and celebrating milestones is essential as it provides a sense of accomplishment and reinforces successful behaviors. Use EFT to enhance these positive feelings. For example, when you complete a significant portion of your goal, like finishing a critical project phase or reaching a fitness milestone, take a moment to tap through the points while focusing on your feelings of achievement. You might use a setup statement such as, "Even though it was challenging, I have successfully completed this phase, and I feel proud and motivated to continue." This boosts your morale and conditions you to associate positive emotions with the effort towards your goals, making the journey enjoyable and fulfilling.

This chapter explored various EFT strategies for setting clear, measurable, and value-aligned goals. We delved into how to construct tapping routines to overcome common obstacles like procrastination and fear of failure and how to maintain motivation through the ups and downs of pursuing significant goals.

Additionally, we highlighted the importance of recognizing and celebrating milestones to reinforce a positive mindset and success-oriented behaviors.

As we wrap up this chapter, remember that the journey toward your goals is a dynamic process that requires persistence, resilience, and a positive mindset. EFT offers tools that empower you to navigate this journey confidently and gracefully. Looking ahead, the next chapter will introduce specialized tapping techniques that cater to unique situations and challenges, further expanding your toolkit for personal and professional growth.

SHARE THE POWER OF TAPPING

"The best way to find yourself is to lose yourself in helping others."

— MAHATMA GANDHI

Thank you for joining me on this journey to explore the power of tapping! I hope "Tapping Into Freedom" has helped you feel more balanced and calm and that you've found joy in using this simple yet powerful technique.

If this book has made a difference in your life, I would love to hear about it! Sharing your thoughts in a review can help others discover how tapping can help them, too. When you write a review, you're doing more than just sharing your opinion—you're helping someone else take the first step toward feeling better.

How to Write Your Review:

- Scan the QR code.
- What did you enjoy most about the book?
- Did any part of the tapping process make you feel calmer or happier?
- Was there a specific section that spoke to you?

Writing a review is simple. Your words don't have to be fancy or long. Just share what felt right for you. Your honest experience might be exactly what someone else needs to see to start their journey of healing and growth.

Your experience is invaluable to us. Thank you for your kindness and for being a part of this community.

With gratitude,

Eloise Rose

CHAPTER 7

SPECIALIZED TAPPING TECHNIQUES

Stepping into your kitchen, you pause, noticing the clock indicates late afternoon when cravings usually hit. Your hand hovers over a drawer, a habitual twitch towards the comforting crackle of a chocolate wrapper. But today, let's choose a different path. What if you could tap into a deeper source of satisfaction and control instead of yielding to that impulsive snack? Emotional Freedom Techniques (EFT), or tapping, offer tools for immediate relief and lasting transformations in managing cravings and maintaining healthy eating habits.

7.1 TAPPING FOR EMOTIONAL EATING AND WEIGHT MANAGEMENT

Identifying Emotional Triggers

The journey to overcoming emotional eating begins with understanding the 'why' behind your impulses. Emotional triggers such as stress, boredom, sadness, or even joy can prompt eating behaviors more about emotional needs than physical hunger. To identify these triggers, remember moments when you find yourself reaching for food unnecessarily. Is it during work pressure, after an upsetting call, or perhaps late at night out of loneliness? Recognizing these patterns is the first step. Once identified, tapping provides a method to manage and transform these impulses.

Using EFT, you can address the emotional roots of your eating habits by tapping on specific points that help release the emotional hold of these triggers. For instance, if stress is a trigger, tapping on the points along the side of the hand (also known as the Karate Chop point) while acknowledging your feelings can help reduce the immediate stress, replacing it with a sense of calm and control over your choices.

Tapping Scripts for Cravings

Crafting effective tapping scripts is essential in managing cravings. These scripts should directly address the craving, emotional undercurrents, and reinforce your self-control. Here's how you might structure a tapping session for cravings:

- Start by addressing the craving: "Even though I have this strong craving for chocolate, I deeply and completely accept myself."
- Tap through the points, acknowledging underlying feelings: "This craving might be about feeling lonely or bored."
- Reinforce self-control as you conclude the sequence: "I choose to find other ways to comfort myself."

This method helps acknowledge the craving without judgment, understand the emotion driving it, and actively choose a healthier response.

Integrating Mindful Eating with EFT

Mindful eating is about being fully present with your eating experience, engaging all senses, and listening to your body's hunger and fullness signals. Integrating mindful eating with EFT can significantly enhance awareness and control over eating behaviors. Start by tapping to clear any emotional or mental clutter before a meal. A simple setup could be, "Even though I usually rush through my meals, I choose to eat mindfully and enjoy each bite." This primes your mind for a more attentive and enjoyable eating experience. During the meal, pause to tap lightly if you notice old habits creeping in, using short reminder phrases like "stay present."

Success Stories and Motivation Outcomes

Hearing from others who have successfully used EFT to manage their weight and emotional eating can be incredibly motivating. Take Clara, for example, who struggled with nightly ice cream binges triggered by stress and loneliness. Through EFT, she learned to manage her emotions differently and gradually replaced binging with healthier habits. Within months, not only did her weight stabilize, but her overall stress levels and emotional well-being improved dramatically. Stories like Clara's illustrate the transformative potential of EFT, providing real-life inspiration for those embarking on similar journeys.

Reflection Section

Take a moment to reflect on your eating behaviors:

- When do you notice yourself eating out of emotion rather than hunger?
- How could tapping help you address these moments?

Jot down your thoughts and any insights that arise. This reflection can be a foundation for your personalized EFT practice in managing emotional eating and weight.

In this chapter, we delve into the specialized technique of tapping not just as a method of crisis management but as a transformative tool for long-term lifestyle changes. As you learn to apply these techniques, the control you gain extends beyond your diet, influencing a broader spectrum of emotional regulation and self-care practices, paving the way towards a healthier, more aware self.

7.2 ADVANCED TAPPING: ADDRESSING MULTIPLE ISSUES SIMULTANEOUSLY

Tapping, or Emotional Freedom Techniques (EFT), often involves addressing a single issue within a session. However, life is rarely so neat, and you might face emotions and challenges that need simultaneous attention. Advanced tapping techniques enable you to navigate multiple issues without feeling overwhelmed, ensuring a harmonious integration of scripts catering to complex emotional states. Here's how you can layer different tapping scripts to effectively address intertwined issues such as stress and insomnia, a combination that many find themselves dealing with concurrently.

When layering tapping scripts, the key is identifying the common emotional thread that links the issues you are experiencing. For instance, stress often exacerbates insomnia and vice versa. Begin by crafting a setup statement that acknowledges both problems, such as, "Even though I am stressed about my work, and it is affecting my sleep, I deeply and completely accept myself and choose to find peace and rest." By acknowledging both stress and insomnia, you set the stage for a tapping session that addresses the root of each issue without diluting the effectiveness of the treatment for either. As you tap through the points, alternate your focus between stress-related phrases and sleep-related phrases. This could look like tapping on the eyebrow point while focusing on stress, "This stress at work," and tapping on the side of the eye while shifting focus to insomnia, "I choose to relax and prepare for restful sleep." This method ensures that both issues are addressed in a single session, promoting a holistic healing process.

Balancing complex emotional states during such sessions is crucial. It's common to feel a surge of emotions when tapping, especially when dealing with multiple issues. To maintain emotional equilibrium throughout the process, use tapping to ground yourself. If emotions become too intense, pause at the heart point at the center of the chest and perform a few taps while breathing deeply. This point is associated with calming the heart and balancing emotions. Remind yourself of your intent to heal and restore balance, using affirmations like, "I am calm and centered, and I handle my emotions with grace."

Prioritizing issues is another critical aspect of advanced tapping. While it can be tempting to tackle all problems at once, prioritizing them based on urgency and impact can enhance the effectiveness of your tapping sessions. Start by listing the issues you face, then assess which ones cause the most disruption in your daily life. For example, if lack of sleep makes it difficult for you to function at work, you might prioritize insomnia over a less pressing concern. Once prioritized, dedicate the initial part of your tapping session to the most pressing issue, using more rounds of tapping to soothe it before moving on to less critical concerns. This strategic approach ensures that the most disruptive issues are given adequate attention and energy, leading to more effective and satisfying outcomes.

Developing advanced reminder phrases is essential in sessions dealing with multiple concerns. These phrases should be concise yet comprehensive enough to encapsulate the nuances of each issue. For example, a reminder phrase like, "Releasing this work stress and embracing calm, restful nights" integrates stress and insomnia into a cohesive focus for tapping. By crafting such phrases, you guide your mind to address each issue within the broader context of your emotional health, reinforcing the interconnectedness of your experiences and the holistic nature of your healing journey.

In applying these advanced tapping techniques, you not only increase the scope of issues you can address in a single session but also enhance your ability to manage complex emotional landscapes. This approach fosters a deeper understanding of the interplay between different aspects of your life. It empowers you to take control of your emotional well-being in a structured, effective manner. As you continue to practice these techniques, you'll likely discover a greater capacity for self-healing and an increased resilience against life's challenges, paving the way for a more balanced, fulfilling life.

7.3 TAPPING TECHNIQUES FOR RELATIONSHIP ISSUES

In the intricate dance of romantic, familial, or platonic relationships, the steps can sometimes become misaligned, leading to missteps and stumbles that disrupt the harmony. Emotional Freedom Techniques (EFT), or tapping, offers a method to retrace these steps, understand the underlying rhythms, and restore the synchrony needed for a smooth and supportive relationship dance. The first step in this process involves mapping out your relationship dynamics. This means looking honestly at how interactions unfold, what emotional patterns emerge, and where conflicts typically arise. It's like sketching a map of a well-traveled road, noting the spots where you frequently hit bumps or encounter detours. By identifying these patterns, you can use EFT to specifically target and address the emotional undercurrents contributing to relationship challenges.

Mapping out relationship dynamics requires you to observe and reflect on your interactions. Consider recent conversations or situations that led to feelings of discomfort or conflict. What emotions were triggered in you? Frustration, sadness, perhaps a sense of being misunderstood? Recognizing these emotional patterns is crucial because it sets the foundation for effective tapping sessions. For each pattern identified, you can create tailored tapping scripts that address these emotional triggers, helping to diffuse them before they escalate into more significant issues.

Once you understand the emotional landscape of your relationships, the next step is to enhance communication and empathy through targeted tapping routines. These routines are designed to open up new communication channels and deepen understanding between parties. For instance, if your discussions often become arguments because each person feels unheard, a tapping script might focus on opening oneself to listen and understand the other's perspective. A possible setup statement could be, "Even though I feel unheard, and it makes me defensive, I choose to listen openly and understand deeply." As you tap through the points, focus on releasing any defensive barriers and invite a sense of openness and empathy. This practice helps in the moment and gradually transforms how you approach conversations, making them more constructive and supportive.

Handling conflicts effectively is another critical aspect of maintaining healthy relationships. When managed poorly, conflicts can lead to lasting resentment and emotional distance. However, tapping offers a tool to handle these situations with more composure and clarity. When a conflict arises, it's easy to get caught up in the heat of the moment, but if you can take a step back and tap, even briefly, it can change the trajectory of the interaction. Start by excusing yourself for a quick moment to tap on the karate chop point, a discreet yet effective point for managing acute stress. Use a setup statement like, "Even though I'm upset and angry right now, I choose to calm down and approach this situation calmly." This helps to reset your emotional state, allowing you to return to the conversation with a cooler head and a more balanced perspective, facilitating a resolution that respects both parties' needs and feelings.

Finally, regular tapping should be considered a vital maintenance tool for any relationship. Just as you might take your car for regular tune-ups to keep it running smoothly, regular tapping can help maintain the health and resilience of your relationship. Set aside time each week to tap on any minor issues that have arisen or general feelings of gratitude and appreciation for your relationship. This prevents minor issues from growing into more significant problems and strengthens the emotional bonds between you and your loved ones. These sessions can be done individually or together, creating a shared space for emotional care and connection.

Incorporating these tapping techniques into your relationship care routine can significantly enhance the quality and depth of your interactions. By actively addressing and managing emotional patterns, improving communication, handling conflicts wisely, and maintaining regular emotional upkeep, you and your loved ones can enjoy a more harmonious and fulfilling relationship. As you continue to apply these strategies, you'll likely find that not only do your relationships improve, but your overall emotional intelligence and capacity for empathy also grow, enriching your life profoundly.

7.4 EFT FOR PROFESSIONAL AND WORKPLACE STRESS

In today's fast-paced professional environments, stress can seem as commonplace as coffee breaks and email notifications. Stress can significantly hinder your productivity and well-being, whether it's a looming deadline, a pile of unmanageable workloads, or navigating complex relationships with colleagues. Recognizing specific sources of workplace stress is the first step toward managing them effectively. For instance, if deadlines constantly have you on edge, acknowledging this can help you tailor your Emotional Freedom Techniques (EFT) sessions to address this trigger specifically. Similarly, interpersonal conflicts with a team member or a supervisor might be your stress catalyst, and pinpointing this can direct your tapping strategies more effectively.

Once you've identified these stressors, the next step is to develop tapping scripts that can be easily applied in your workplace. These scripts must be discreet yet effective, allowing quick relief without drawing unnecessary attention. For example, suppose you're feeling overwhelmed by a project. You might step aside for a few minutes and use a simple tapping script like, "Even though I feel overwhelmed by this project, I accept myself and my feelings, and I choose to find clarity and focus." You can tap discreetly at your desk or in a quiet corner. Using the side of the hand or tapping under the eye are subtle yet effective points that can be tapped without drawing much attention.

Improving professional relationships is another crucial area where EFT can be remarkably effective. Workplace environments often require us to navigate a maze of relationships, including those with direct reports, peers, and superiors. These relationships can have challenges, such as authority conflicts with a superior or collaboration issues within a team. EFT can help address these problems by reducing the stress they cause and opening up new pathways for empathy and understanding. A tapping script in this context might look like, "Even though I feel frustrated with my team, I deeply and completely accept myself and choose to approach our interactions with openness and understanding." This approach encourages a shift from a reactive emotional state to one of proactive problem-solving.

Building resilience in high-pressure environments is one of the most significant benefits EFT offers professionals. High-pressure situations are not just about the immediate stressors; they also test our long-term capacity to cope with stress. Tapping can be a powerful tool in these scenarios, helping to build and maintain resilience over time. Techniques focusing on building resilience might involve tapping on future-oriented affirmations like, "I am capable of handling pressure gracefully and efficiently." This helps in the moment and fortifies your psychological resilience, preparing you for future challenges.

EFT offers a practical and accessible tool to manage workplace stress, enhance professional relationships, and build resilience. Applying these techniques can improve your immediate work environment and contribute to a more fulfilling and productive career. As we close this chapter, remember that stress does not have to be an inevitable part of your work life. With EFT, you have the power to transform how you experience and manage stress, leading to a more enjoyable and successful professional life. The next chapter will explore how EFT can be adapted for special populations, expanding the scope of this powerful tool to meet diverse needs and situations.

CHAPTER 8

INTEGRATING EFT INTO DAILY LIFE

Imagine your typical day as a bustling city where each task and interaction contributes to the hustle and bustle. Now, think of EFT, or Emotional Freedom Techniques, as your personal sanctuary within this city—a quiet space where you can retreat to regroup and recharge. Integrating EFT into your daily life isn't just about managing moments of stress; it's about transforming your everyday experience and making peace and clarity more accessible, no matter the chaos around you. This chapter will guide you through designing a daily tapping routine tailored to your unique lifestyle, helping you harness the restorative power of EFT from morning to night.

8.1 DESIGNING YOUR DAILY TAPPING ROUTINE

Assessing Daily Needs and Stressors

To integrate EFT into your life effectively, conduct a thoughtful assessment of your daily schedule. Identify specific times or situations where stress tends to accumulate. Is it during the morning rush, the midday slump, or perhaps in the evening when you're winding down? Understanding these patterns is crucial as it allows you to strategically place tapping sessions where they will be most beneficial. For instance, if you notice that your stress peaks in the mid-afternoon, that might be the ideal time for a brief tapping break.

This assessment isn't just about recognizing when you feel stressed but understanding what triggers these feelings. Are these triggers related to specific activities, interactions, or certain times of the day? Pinpointing these details will enhance your ability to manage stress proactively with EFT. It's like mapping out the terrain of your day and marking the rough patches—once you know where they are, you can navigate them more smoothly.

Customizable Tapping Plans

With a clear understanding of when and why you tend to feel stressed, you can begin to create a tapping routine that addresses your specific needs. Think of this as creating a series of small sanctuaries throughout your day. A brief tapping session focused on setting a positive tone for the day can be incredibly effective for morning energization. Incorporate affirmations related to energy and focus, such as "I am filled with energy and ready for the day ahead."

Consider a routine that helps recalibrate your mood and focus for midday stress relief. This might involve tapping on points that alleviate stress and enhance clarity, accompanied by affirmations like "I release this stress and welcome calmness." In the evening, a routine aimed at relaxation can help you unwind. Here, your tapping might focus on letting go of the day's burdens, using affirmations such as "I let go of today's stresses and embrace peaceful rest."

Integration with Daily Activities

To ensure that EFT becomes a natural part of your day, look for opportunities to integrate it into activities you're already doing. For example, while waiting for your morning coffee to brew, use those few minutes for a quick tapping session. Or, while lunch is heating up, tap away any tension from the morning. These small integrations can make a big difference, helping to keep stress at bay and ensuring that tapping doesn't feel like another task on your to-do list.

Tracking Progress and Adjustments

Finally, to truly tailor your routine to your evolving needs, make a habit of tracking your progress. Use a journal or an app to note how you feel before and after tapping. This record-keeping will not only provide you with insight into how effective your routines are but also help you fine-tune them. You may find that tapping in the morning tremendously impacts your day, or you may discover that a quick session before an important meeting helps maintain your focus. By keeping track of these outcomes, you can continuously optimize your tapping routines, making them more effective and personalized over time.

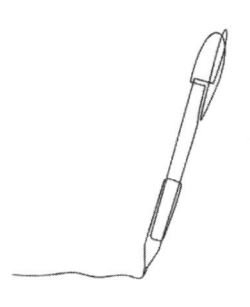

By assessing your daily needs, customizing your tapping plans, integrating EFT into your regular activities, and tracking your progress, you can create a tapping routine that addresses your current stressors and evolves with you, providing support and relief as your life changes and grows. This approach ensures that EFT isn't just a technique you turn to in times of crisis but a consistent, nurturing presence in your life, helping you navigate each day with more ease and resilience.

8.2 TAPPING WHILE TRAVELING: TECHNIQUES ON THE GO

Traveling, whether for leisure or business, often brings its own set of challenges and stressors. From the discomfort of cramped airplane seats to the anxiety of navigating unfamiliar places, these situations can disrupt our emotional balance and trigger stress responses. Integrating Emotional Freedom Techniques (EFT), or tapping, into your travel routine can be a game-changer, offering a portable method to manage stress and enhance your travel experience. This section explores practical strategies for incorporating tapping into your travels, ensuring that you have tools at your disposal to maintain calm and composure no matter where you are.

Tapping During Commutes

Commuting, especially in crowded conditions such as buses, trains, or planes, can often feel like a test of patience and endurance. To integrate tapping discreetly during these times, focus on simple, easily accessible tapping points that are less noticeable to others. The side of the hand, also known as the karate chop point, is an excellent spot for this purpose. This point can be tapped gently with the fingers of the other hand, all while appearing as if you are merely resting your hands in your lap or adjusting your grip on your seat. Another subtle tapping point is the collarbone point, which can be accessed by crossing your arms over your chest, mimicking a casual pose, and tapping gently. These techniques allow you to tap without drawing attention, calming your nerves and reducing stress levels discreetly.

Adapting your tapping script to fit the context of your commute can also enhance its effectiveness. For instance, if you are getting impatient with the pace of traffic or the noise level on a train, your setup statement could be, "Even though I feel irritated by this noise, I deeply and completely accept myself and choose to feel calm." Repeat this or a similar affirmation while tapping the accessible points, using the rhythm of the tapping to soothe your frustration and help refocus your mind on something more positive.

Handling Travel Anxiety

Travel anxiety, including the fear of flying or anxiety about being in unfamiliar environments, is common and can significantly impact your travel experience. To address this, specific tapping techniques tailored to these fears can be beneficial. Before your trip, practice tapping sequences that address your particular anxieties. For example, if flying is a stressor, tap to work through your fears days before your flight. Your setup statement might be, "Even though I'm scared of flying, I deeply and completely accept myself and trust that I am safe." As you tap through the points, visualize yourself traveling calmly and confidently.

During your travels, keep this script handy for quick access. Excuse yourself to a restroom or another private space and run through your tapping routine if anxiety arises. This can help reset your emotional state, reduce anxiety, and allow you to continue your journey more easily. Remember, the key is repetition and consistency; the more you practice tapping in response to travel anxiety, the more natural and effective it mitigates stress.

Quick and Effective Tapping Scripts

For travelers, having quick and effective tapping scripts is essential. These scripts should be tailored to common travel stressors and designed to quickly bring about a sense of calm. Develop a few go-to phrases you can easily remember and apply in various situations. For instance, a general script for travel-related stress might be, "Even though I feel overwhelmed right now, I choose to be calm and centered." This can be used in various scenarios, from dealing with lost luggage to navigating a busy tourist attraction.

To make these scripts as effective as possible, practice them regularly during less stressful times so that they come to mind quickly when you really need them. This preparation makes it more likely that you'll use tapping effectively when travel stress hits, providing quick relief and helping you regain your composure.

Portable Tapping Tools

To facilitate tapping while traveling, consider creating portable tools that assist in your practice. Tapping point cards are a great option, as they can be small enough to fit in your wallet or pocket. These cards can feature diagrams of tapping points and sample affirmations or scripts, serving as a quick reference in moments of stress. Additionally, several mobile apps guide users through tapping sequences and provide customizable options for different situations, including travel. These apps can be beneficial as they often come with features that allow you to track your sessions and mood over time, helping you gauge the effectiveness of your tapping practice as you travel.

By adopting these strategies, tapping becomes a therapeutic tool and a travel companion that supports your emotional well-being on the go. Whether you're navigating the challenges of a daily commute or the complexities of international travel, EFT provides a practical, effective way to manage stress and enhance your overall travel experience, making every journey more enjoyable and relaxed.

8.3 INCORPORATING TAPPING INTO MORNING AND EVENING ROUTINES

Starting your day with a positive mindset and ending it with a sense of calm can significantly enhance your overall well-being. Integrating Emotional Freedom Techniques (EFT), or tapping, into your morning and evening routines helps establish these beneficial states, setting the tone for productive days and refreshing nights. Here's how you can embed this powerful practice into the bookends of your day, ensuring you begin and conclude in harmony and balance.

Morning Tapping for a Positive Start

Imagine waking up, feeling the weight of yesterday's unresolved issues or the daunting tasks of the day ahead. Instead of carrying this burden, you can use tapping to set a positive tone for the day. Begin by finding a quiet moment after you wake up. Before you check your phone or start your daily chores, take a few minutes for a tapping session. Focus on clearing any residual negativity or anxiety from the previous day or any apprehension about the day ahead. For example, your setup statement might be, "Even though I feel overwhelmed about today, I deeply and completely accept myself and choose to embrace positivity." As you tap through the points, visualize yourself handling the day's challenges calmly and confidently. Embed affirmations that reinforce this imagery, such as "I am capable and ready to tackle today's tasks with ease and joy." This practice helps dissipate morning anxiety and invigorate your spirit, equipping you with a mindset of efficiency and positivity.

Evening Tapping for Relaxation and Reflection

After a day filled with activities and interactions, your mind and body need to unwind and process the day's events. Creating an evening tapping routine aids in transitioning from daytime busyness to nighttime relaxation. This routine can be particularly effective right before you begin your bedtime rituals. Taping is used to reflect on the day, acknowledging both successes and challenges. Your setup statement might be something like, "Even though I had a tough day, I deeply and completely accept myself and choose to release this stress." Focus on letting go of specific stresses or general tension. Incorporate affirmations that promote relaxation, such as "I allow myself to relax deeply and completely now." This helps alleviate stress and prepares your mind for restful sleep, processing and releasing the day's emotional residue.

Tapping to Improve Sleep Quality

Sleep issues, such as insomnia or a restless mind, can significantly impact your life, affecting everything from your mood to your productivity. Tapping can be a valuable tool in your arsenal to combat these issues. Develop a specific tapping routine aimed at promoting sleep. Start this routine as part of your bedtime ritual, perhaps after you've dimmed the lights and before you get into bed. Target common concerns that keep you awake, like racing thoughts or anxiety about upcoming events. Your setup statement could be, "Even though I feel too anxious to sleep, I deeply and completely accept myself and choose to feel calm and sleepy." As you tap, focus on calming the mind and body, encouraging a state conducive to sleep. Phrases like "I welcome sleep" or "My mind is calm and quiet" can be effective. Over time, this routine can help realign your natural sleep rhythms, improving the quality and duration of your sleep.

Consistency for Habit Formation

Consistency is the key to reaping the full benefits of tapping into your morning and evening routines. Make tapping a non-negotiable part of your daily schedule, like brushing your teeth or having meals. Consistency helps solidify these practices as habits, embedding them deeply within your daily rhythm. To build this consistency, set reminders for yourself at first. Place sticky notes on your bathroom mirror or set alarms on your phone as prompts to tap. Over time, as tapping becomes ingrained in your daily routine, you'll find that it naturally blends into your day without the need for reminders. This habitual practice ensures that you regularly clear emotional debris and maintain a state of mental clarity, significantly enhancing your overall quality of life and well-being.

Integrating tapping into your morning and evening routines creates powerful bookends for your day, ensuring you start and end on positive, calm notes. This practice enhances your immediate mental and emotional state and contributes to long-term health and happiness, proving that a few minutes of tapping can transform your entire day.

8.4 USING TAPPING TO MAINTAIN EMOTIONAL BALANCE THROUGHOUT THE DAY

Maintaining emotional balance in the ebb and flow of daily life is akin to walking a tightrope. It requires focus, adaptability, and a set of strategies to stay centered amid the unexpected gusts of wind that represent day-to-day stressors and emotional disturbances. The practice of Emotional Freedom Techniques (EFT), or tapping, offers a dynamic approach to managing these fluctuations. By developing responsive tapping strategies, you can quickly recalibrate your emotional state, ensuring minor disturbances don't escalate into major disruptions.

Responsive tapping strategies are about having a toolkit of quick, effective techniques ready to deploy at a moment's notice. Consider this: you're about to give a critical presentation, and suddenly, nerves strike. Instead of letting anxiety derail your performance, a brief tapping session can help realign your emotions, boosting confidence and calm. Start by identifying a 'go-to' point that feels most effective for you—many find the collarbone point to be discreet and easy to access. Pair this with a simple affirmation like, "I am calm and in control." This quick intervention can be done almost anywhere, from a busy office to the quiet of a bathroom stall, allowing you to manage your emotions without needing a significant break from your activities.

Preventative tapping techniques can be invaluable for those who often face high-stress situations, whether in personal or professional settings. These involve using EFT before you step into known stress-inducing scenarios to fortify your emotional resilience. For instance, a proactive tapping session can prepare you mentally and emotionally if you have a challenging meeting on your schedule. You might use affirmations such as, "I handle stressful situations with grace and effectiveness," while tapping through the EFT points. This prepares you to handle the upcoming stressor more effectively and helps you gradually reprogramme your response to such situations.

The highs and lows of emotions aren't just about external events; they also reflect our internal responses and conditionings. Balancing these emotional highs and lows through tapping involves acknowledging and addressing both extremes. If you find yourself overly excited or excessively down, tapping can help modulate these feelings. Use tapping to explore these emotional states deeply—ask yourself what's driving these feelings, tap on recognizing these emotions, and use affirmations to bring yourself to a state of equilibrium. Phrases like "I embrace my emotions and guide them towards balance" can be powerful. This conscious regulation helps maintain a more stable emotional state, which supports better decision-making and interpersonal interactions throughout the day.

Incorporating mindfulness with tapping enhances the effectiveness of both practices. Mindfulness, the art of being present and fully engaged with the now, without overreaction or overwhelming emotion, complements EFT's physical and cognitive aspects. By integrating mindfulness into your tapping sessions, you focus intensely on each tap, each breath, and each affirmation. This deepens your awareness of the present moment and your current emotional state, allowing for more profound and lasting shifts. For example, as you tap on the eyebrow point, intensely focus on the sensation of your fingertips on your skin, the sound of your affirmation, and the rhythm of your breath. This integration enriches your tapping practice and cultivates a mindfulness habit that can extend beyond structured sessions into everyday life activities.

By weaving these strategies into the fabric of your daily routine, you ensure that tapping isn't just a reactive tool but a proactive approach to cultivating and maintaining emotional balance. This ongoing practice enhances your ability to handle the day's challenges and contributes to long-term emotional health and resilience.

As this chapter closes, we reflect on the transformative potential of integrating EFT into daily life. Tapping is a versatile and powerful tool, from enhancing morning routines to ensuring calm evenings, managing travel stress, and maintaining emotional balance throughout the day. It is my hope that these strategies not only serve you in moments of need but become integral practices that enhance your overall quality of life. The next chapter will explore overcoming common challenges and objections associated with EFT, further empowering you to optimize and personalize your tapping experience.

CHAPTER 9
OVERCOMING COMMON CHALLENGES AND OBJECTIONS

Imagine approaching a small, unassuming door you've walked past countless times. Today, with a key called EFT, you decide to see what's on the other side. As the door creaks open, you're met with a room of mirrors, each reflecting an exaggerated, funhouse version of yourself. This is the room of your unexamined fears and doubts about trying something new, like tapping. Just as you might initially feel out of place in this strange, mirrored room, beginning EFT can make you feel self-conscious or even silly. But remember, every expert in anything was once a beginner, feeling out of place as they took their first tentative steps. This chapter guides you through that room, turning the funhouse into a corridor of clear, reassuring reflections affirming your journey with EFT.

9.1 "I FEEL SILLY TAPPING": OVERCOMING SELF-CONSCIOUSNESS

The feeling of silliness while tapping is a common initial hurdle. It's a natural reaction, especially when trying an approach involving tapping your body while speaking affirmations out loud. It's essential to recognize that this feeling is a normal part of the process experienced by many beginners. When you first begin to tap, it can seem strange to think that tapping specific points on your body could alter your emotional state. This skepticism is compounded by the fear of how it looks or sounds to others who might not understand your actions. However, embracing this stage is crucial; it's where growth begins.

To ease into the practice of EFT, start in a private space where you feel secure and free from judgment. This could be a quiet room in your home or even a secluded spot in nature. Begin with simple, short sessions focusing on noticeable stressors that don't feel overwhelming. As you notice the benefits—perhaps a sense of relief after tapping or a sudden clarity about a problem—your confidence in the process will grow. Gradually, as your comfort increases, you might extend your tapping sessions or even integrate them into your daily routine, possibly before a workday begins or in a car before entering a social event.

Shifting your focus to the outcomes rather than the process itself can also significantly reduce feelings of self-consciousness. For instance, if you're tapping to alleviate anxiety, concentrate on the relief and calmness that follow your sessions. Celebrating these small victories can reinforce the effectiveness of EFT and motivate you to continue. It helps to set realistic, measurable goals at the start of your EFT journey, such as reducing panic attack frequency from daily to weekly and tracking these changes. By focusing on these tangible benefits, you validate the process internally, making it easier to integrate tapping into your life without feeling self-conscious.

Sharing Success Stories

Hearing from others who once stood where you are now can be incredibly reassuring. Consider the story of Tom, a client who initially felt foolish as he tapped on his forehead, thinking, "How could this help?" Yet, with persistence, he experienced significant relief from chronic insomnia. Tom shared how he went from feeling embarrassed to openly discussing EFT with friends and family, many of whom were curious and eventually eager to try it themselves after seeing his transformation. These stories are a powerful reminder that while the start might be bumpy, persistence is key, and the results can be profoundly life-changing.

Stories like Tom's are not rare; they are among the myriad experiences of individuals who initially felt silly but found great relief and success through EFT. These narratives form a collective testament to the efficacy and transformative potential of tapping, providing both inspiration and a sense of community to those starting their EFT practice. They serve as a bridge, connecting the initial discomfort to a place of confidence and advocacy for the practice. They illustrate that the journey through self-consciousness leads to a rewarding destination of emotional freedom and self-discovery.

9.2 DEALING WITH SKEPTICISM: HOW TO RESPOND TO DOUBTERS

When you first share your experiences with Emotional Freedom Techniques (EFT), you might encounter skepticism from friends, family, or colleagues. It's a natural response, especially for those unfamiliar with EFT's principles. Skepticism isn't just a barrier; it's an invitation to deepen your understanding and articulate the value of your practice more clearly. Part of incorporating EFT into your life is learning how to address doubts gracefully—both your own and others—with patience and evidence.

Arming yourself with facts is a powerful strategy. The efficacy of EFT has been the subject of numerous studies that provide empirical support for its benefits. For instance, research published in the *Journal of Psychological Health* found that EFT significantly decreased depression and anxiety scores among participants. Another *Journal of Alternative and Complementary Medicine* study reported that EFT helped reduce psychological stress and improve immune system functioning. When discussing EFT with skeptics, citing such studies can help shift the conversation from subjective opinion to one grounded in research. It's beneficial to explain how EFT works, perhaps likening it to acupuncture but without needles, to help others understand the method's basis in established practices like Chinese medicine's meridian system.

Sharing personal experiences can also be incredibly persuasive. Stories resonate profoundly and can often bridge the gap between doubt and openness. You might share how EFT helped you overcome a long-standing phobia or how it has been instrumental in managing your stress levels. Personal anecdotes about how tapping before a significant event helped maintain your calm or improve your focus can illustrate the practical benefits of EFT in everyday life. Encourage others who have seen positive results from EFT to share their stories, too. Sometimes, hearing about a familiar person's successful experience can be more convincing than any scientific study.

Inviting skeptics to try EFT for themselves can be a turning point. Suggest starting with something small and non-threatening, like using EFT to handle the stress of a busy day or to manage minor aches and pains. Offer to guide them through their first few tapping sessions, providing a safe and supportive environment for their initial experience. This direct experience often dispels myths and misconceptions about EFT more effectively than any explanation. It turns abstract concepts into personal experiences, which can be a powerful catalyst for changing opinions.

Lastly, it's crucial to respect differences in opinion. EFT may not resonate with everyone like any other practice, and that's okay. Learning when to engage and when to step back is part of using EFT wisely. If someone remains skeptical despite your best efforts, respect their viewpoint and focus on your own path. EFT is a personal tool for growth and healing; its value for you does not diminish if others view it differently. Maintaining this perspective helps preserve relationships and keeps your practice focused on personal well-being rather than external validation.

Navigating skepticism requires a balance of education, personal testimony, and openness to others' viewpoints. By confidently sharing your knowledge and experiences and inviting others to have their own, you defend your practice and possibly open up a new avenue of healing for someone else. Remember, each conversation about EFT, whether it leads to acceptance or not, is an opportunity to refine your understanding and enhance your communication skills, which are integral parts of your growth journey with EFT.

9.3 WHEN TAPPING DOESN'T WORK: TROUBLESHOOTING COMMON ISSUES

Sometimes, despite your best efforts, it may feel like Emotional Freedom Techniques (EFT) needs to be fixed. It's easy to feel discouraged when the results aren't immediate or as impactful as anticipated. However, this is often a crucial moment for learning and adjustment rather than a sign that EFT isn't suitable for you. Let's explore some effective strategies to troubleshoot and enhance your tapping practice.

Firstly, it's essential to review your tapping technique. EFT is quite precise—where and how you tap matters. Each tapping point corresponds to specific meridians in the body, and incorrect tapping can dilute the effectiveness of your practice. Start by ensuring that you are tapping lightly yet firmly. The pressure should be enough to feel a slight drumming sensation but not so hard that it feels uncomfortable.

Additionally, each point should be tapped approximately five to seven times before moving to the next. If you're new to EFT or have been self-taught, revisiting instructional videos or diagrams might be helpful to ensure your technique is correct. Sometimes, even experienced practitioners find it beneficial to refresh their knowledge of the tapping points and sequences to maintain the efficacy of their practice.

Adjusting expectations is another key aspect of a sustainable EFT practice. Emotional and physical issues vary in complexity and intensity, as does the time it takes to address them through EFT. Some issues may see immediate relief after a few sessions, while deeper or more chronic problems require persistent effort. It's crucial to set realistic expectations based on the nature of the issue you're addressing. For example, if you're dealing with long-standing anxiety, it's reasonable to expect gradual improvement rather than immediate relief. Consistency is your ally here. Regular tapping, even on days when you feel better, helps reinforce the gains you've made and prevents backsliding.

Exploring underlying issues is one of the most profound aspects of EFT. Often, when progress seems stalled, it's because the surface issue you're addressing is a symptom of a deeper, unresolved problem. For instance, difficulty in managing anger might be rooted in unresolved trauma from past experiences that you might not have consciously connected to your current emotional responses. In such cases, merely tapping on anger might bring temporary relief but won't address the root cause. Here, delving deeper into your emotional history, with the guidance of a journal or a therapist, can help identify these foundational issues. Once identified, you can tailor your EFT sessions to target these deeper problems, potentially leading to more significant and lasting changes.

Lastly, seeking professional guidance can dramatically improve your EFT experience, especially when self-administered tapping doesn't seem to yield results. An experienced EFT practitioner can offer personalized guidance tailored to your emotional needs. They can help fine-tune your tapping technique, suggest modifications to your scripts, and aid in uncovering and addressing deeper emotional issues. Professional EFT practitioners also provide the support and encouragement that can be crucial when dealing with challenging emotions or when you feel stuck. If you think that your progress with EFT has plateaued or if specific issues feel too overwhelming to handle alone, consider scheduling a session with a certified EFT therapist. Their expertise can provide new insights and directions, enriching your practice and enhancing its effectiveness.

By systematically addressing these areas—refining your technique, setting realistic expectations, exploring more profound issues, and seeking professional input—you can maximize the effectiveness of your EFT practice and overcome the hurdles that might currently seem insurmountable. These steps help make EFT more effective and deepen your understanding of your emotional landscape, empowering you to manage your emotional well-being more proactively and confidently.

9.4 MAINTAINING MOTIVATION: WHAT TO DO WHEN PROGRESS SLOWS DOWN

Staying motivated can be one of the biggest hurdles in any personal development practice, including Emotional Freedom Techniques (EFT). It's common to encounter moments when it feels like your progress has plateaued or when the initial enthusiasm wanes. Setting small, achievable goals within your EFT practice is crucial to navigating these periods effectively. These goals act like stepping stones across a river—they keep you moving forward, even when the current feels strong. For instance, instead of aiming to eliminate all anxiety, you might set a goal to manage the anxiety you feel during work meetings. This smaller, more specific goal is more manageable and provides a clear target on which to focus your tapping sessions. As you achieve these smaller goals, they accumulate, leading to significant improvements over time that might not have been noticeable if you were only looking for one significant change.

Celebrating every small victory is equally essential. Each time you notice a reduction in your stress level after tapping or when you successfully use EFT to calm yourself in a situation that would have previously upset you, take a moment to acknowledge this progress. No matter how minor they seem, these victories are concrete evidence that your efforts are paying off. They serve as important motivational boosts, reinforcing the value of your continued practice. You might even choose to celebrate these moments in special ways, such as treating yourself to a favorite activity or simply reflecting on your journey and the strides you've made.

Introducing variety into your tapping routines can also significantly enhance your motivation. This could mean changing your scripts, tapping on different issues, or altering your environment —perhaps by tapping outdoors or in a different room. Freshness in practice keeps the process engaging and prevents it from becoming monotonous. For example, if you've been focusing heavily on tapping for stress, you might switch your focus to tapping for creativity or physical well-being. This revitalizes your interest and might lead you to discover new benefits of tapping that you hadn't considered before.

Connecting with the EFT community is another powerful way to sustain motivation. Whether online or in person, these communities offer invaluable support and insight. They provide a platform to share experiences and learn from others on similar paths. Hearing how others have overcome their challenges with EFT can be incredibly inspiring and reassuring. It reminds you that persistence pays off and you are not alone in your struggles. Many find that sharing their stories and successes in these communities bolsters their motivation and helps others, creating a positive reinforcement and support cycle.

These strategies, though simple, can profoundly impact your ability to maintain motivation and continue reaping the benefits of EFT. You keep your practice alive and dynamic by setting achievable goals, celebrating small victories, varying your routines, and engaging with the community. Each of these elements plays a crucial role in building a sustainable and rewarding EFT practice that continues to evolve and enrich your life.

As we wrap up this chapter on maintaining motivation and overcoming common challenges, remember that every journey will have ebbs and flows. The techniques and insights shared here are designed to empower you to keep moving forward, especially when the going gets tough. The next chapter will explore special populations and considerations, expanding the scope of EFT's applicability and offering new perspectives on how this versatile tool can be adapted to meet a wide range of needs and circumstances.

CHAPTER 10
SPECIAL POPULATIONS AND CONSIDERATIONS

10.1 EFT FOR CHILDREN: TECHNIQUES AND CONSIDERATIONS

Imagine you're introducing a child to the vast and enchanting world of a garden. Each plant and flower, from the towering sunflower to the tiny, vibrant daisy, holds a unique story and a lesson within its roots and leaves. Similarly, introducing Emotional Freedom Techniques (EFT) to children involves translating EFT's complex language and techniques into a more straightforward, more captivating format that resonates with their young minds. This process simplifies and makes each tapping session as engaging and enjoyable as an exploration in that garden.

Simplifying EFT for Younger Minds

Children are naturally imaginative, responding wonderfully to stories and characters that animate their experiences. When introducing EFT to children, it's effective to weave the tapping points into narratives or associate them with favorite characters from cartoons or books. For instance, while tapping on the top of the head, you might say, "Imagine you're wearing a crown like a king or queen, and each tap lets your wisdom shine a little brighter." This makes the process fun and vividly embeds the practice in their memory. Simplifying the language involves using terms and explanations that match their level of understanding, avoiding medical or technical jargon, and instead using metaphors and simple descriptions that relate to their everyday experiences.

Addressing Common Childhood Issues

Children face a myriad of challenges, from school-related anxieties to fears of the dark or difficulties in making friends. Tailoring EFT scripts to these issues involves recognizing the emotional context children can relate to and ensuring the scripts are age-appropriate. For example, a tapping script for school anxiety might involve simple affirmations like, "Even though I feel scared about my test, I am a smart and brave student." This not only helps in reducing their anxiety but also boosts their self-esteem. Similarly, for younger children who might be afraid of the dark, tapping sessions could focus on instilling a sense of safety and control with scripts like, "Even though the night is dark, I am safe in my cozy bed."

Parental Involvement

The role of parents in this process is crucial. Not only do they provide the necessary encouragement and support, but they also act as guides in teaching and supervising the tapping techniques. It's essential for parents to first familiarize themselves with EFT—understanding the basic principles and methods—before introducing them to their children. Parents should approach these sessions with patience and positivity, making each tapping experience a shared bonding activity rather than a chore. Guidelines for parents might include keeping the sessions short to maintain the child's attention and interest and consistently integrating tapping into the child's daily routine, perhaps making it a fun game or a bedtime ritual.

Creating a Safe Emotional Space

One of the most important aspects of practicing EFT with children is creating a safe and supportive environment where they feel free to express their emotions and thoughts. Children need to know that their feelings are valid and that they are heard. This involves active listening, where the parent or caregiver gives their full attention to the child's concerns without judgment or immediate correction. It's about fostering an atmosphere of trust and openness where the child feels comfortable discussing their fears or worries. Ensuring this emotional safety is critical to the effectiveness of EFT, as it empowers the child to fully engage with the tapping process and benefit from its healing potential.

Incorporating EFT into children's lives not only aids in managing their immediate emotional and physical challenges but also equips them with a valuable tool for emotional regulation that can benefit them throughout their lives. By adapting EFT to suit their young minds, involving parents in the process, and ensuring a safe and supportive environment, we can effectively extend the profound benefits of EFT to the younger generation, helping them grow into healthier and happier individuals.

10.2 TAPPING IN ELDERLY CARE: ADAPTATIONS AND BENEFITS

Adapting Tapping for Physical Limitations

As we age, our bodies often present new challenges and limitations that require adaptations in managing our health. Emotional Freedom Techniques (EFT), commonly known as tapping, is no exception to this rule. For older adults, especially those dealing with arthritis, reduced mobility, or other physical constraints, the traditional tapping points might not be easily accessible. However, they can still benefit from this powerful technique; it simply means we must adjust our approach. For instance, if reaching for the top of the head or the feet is difficult, alternative points that offer similar benefits can be used instead. Points like the collarbone or under the arm can be easily accessed and tapped with minimal effort. Moreover, older adults can perform tapping with a lighter touch. The pressure doesn't need to be firm to be effective; gentle tapping is sufficient to stimulate the meridian points and achieve the desired emotional relief. This gentler approach ensures the process remains comfortable and safe, avoiding strain or discomfort.

Addressing Age-Related Concerns

One of the profound benefits of EFT for older people is its ability to address a wide range of age-related concerns. Many older adults deal with complex emotions stemming from significant life changes such as retirement, losing loved ones, or declining health. These are not just mere changes but are profound transitions that can affect one's emotional and physical well-being. Tapping offers a method to work through these emotions gently and effectively. For instance, scripts can be developed to specifically address the grief of losing a spouse or the anxiety that comes with health concerns. A script might include setup statements like, "Even though I am grieving, I deeply and completely accept myself and my feelings," followed by reminder phrases such as "It's okay to feel sad," which are repeated during the tapping sequence. This targeted approach allows individuals to acknowledge their feelings, reduce the intensity of their emotional pain, and find a greater sense of peace and acceptance.

Enhancing Cognitive Function and Emotional Health

Recent studies and case studies have shed light on the benefits of EFT for emotional health and cognitive function among the elderly. Tapping has been shown to improve focus, clarity, and mental alertness, which are often areas of concern as one ages. The stimulation of meridian points in EFT has been linked to increased blood flow and reduced stress levels, which in turn can help enhance cognitive functions. Regular tapping can help maintain a sharper mind and also alleviate feelings of confusion or forgetfulness. Furthermore, the emotional health benefits of EFT are particularly useful in combating the feelings of isolation and loneliness that many elderly individuals experience. By reducing stress and anxiety through tapping, individuals can achieve a better emotional balance, enhancing their overall quality of life.

Integrating with Other Therapies

Integrating EFT with other therapies and care routines commonly used in elderly care settings can provide a holistic approach to health and well-being. For example, EFT can be seamlessly combined with physical therapy exercises to enhance physical and emotional resilience. While a therapist helps with mobility and physical strength, tapping can address any emotional resistance or frustration related to physical limitations or the therapy process. Additionally, in settings where medication is prescribed for anxiety or depression, EFT can be a complementary approach, possibly enhancing the effectiveness of medical treatments and, in some cases, reducing reliance on medications. This integration addresses the physical and emotional aspects of health. It ensures that care for the elderly is comprehensive, considering all facets of well-being in a harmonious and supportive manner.

By adapting tapping techniques to the specific needs and limitations of the elderly, addressing their unique emotional concerns, enhancing their cognitive functions, and integrating EFT with other therapeutic practices, we can significantly improve the quality of care provided to older adults. This holistic approach not only aids in managing health conditions but also enriches the lives of elderly individuals, allowing them to navigate the challenges of aging with greater ease and dignity.

10.3 EFT FOR ATHLETES: ENHANCING PERFORMANCE AND RECOVERY

In the realm of sports, where seconds can separate champions from the rest, the mental game plays a crucial role. Emotional Freedom Techniques (EFT) offer athletes a unique edge, equipping them with tools to enhance performance, expedite recovery, and handle the rollercoaster of competitive emotions. Let's explore how incorporating EFT can transform an athlete's approach to training and competition, pushing the boundaries of what is physically and mentally possible.

Optimizing Performance

Athletic performance is as much about mental preparation as it is about physical training. EFT provides strategies to enhance focus, maintain composure, and overcome performance anxiety, which are essential for athletes under pressure. For instance, consider a swimmer battling pre-race nerves. A tailored EFT script might focus on calming the mind and centering the athlete's energy. Phrases like "Even though I feel nervous, I deeply trust my training and my body's capabilities" can be tapped on points such as the karate chop or under the eye, areas associated with fear and anxiety relief. This helps reduce nervousness and reinforces a positive mindset, which is crucial before stepping onto the starting blocks. Furthermore, visualization combined with tapping can significantly boost performance. Athletes can use EFT to reinforce mental images of success, such as visualizing crossing the finish line first and enhancing the psychological readiness that often dictates performance outcomes.

Speeding Recovery

Recovery is an integral part of any athlete's regimen, crucial for physical repair and mentally preparing for the next challenge. EFT aids in this recovery process by addressing the physical pain and emotional stress that often accompany injuries. Tapping on points related to pain relief and stress, such as the top of the head and the collarbone, while focusing on phrases like "I allow my body to heal and recover fully," can promote faster recovery. The reduction in cortisol levels through tapping also aids in better sleep, enhancing the body's natural healing processes. This approach not only speeds up the physical recovery but also helps maintain a positive outlook during the rehabilitation period, a time when many athletes struggle with frustration and despondence.

Handling Competitive Stress

The pressures of competition can evoke a spectrum of emotions, from the thrill of victory to the agony of defeat. Managing these emotions is pivotal for maintaining performance levels and overall well-being. EFT offers a method to navigate these emotional waters effectively. After a tough loss, tapping on feelings of disappointment and reinforcing resilience can be incredibly beneficial. Scripts like "Even though I lost today, I choose to learn from this experience and grow stronger" help in processing defeat more constructively. Conversely, handling victory with grace is equally important. EFT can help balance emotions by tapping on maintaining humility and focus for future competitions, ensuring that success does not breed complacency.

Routine Integration

Integrating EFT into regular training routines ensures that athletes consistently maintain high levels of performance and well-being. This integration might look like beginning each training session with a round of tapping to set a positive, focused tone for the workout. Similarly, ending sessions with tapping can help wind down and reflect on the training, reinforcing positive takeaways and areas for improvement. Coaches can also incorporate group tapping sessions to enhance team cohesion and collective focus, which is particularly useful in team sports where synergy is pivotal.

For athletes, tapping is not just about improving what they do on the track, court, field, or pool; it's about transforming how they approach their sport mentally and emotionally. It equips them with the tools to enhance performance and forge a more resilient, focused, and balanced athletic career. As more athletes and coaches recognize the benefits of EFT, its integration into sports training and recovery protocols continues to expand, promising a new era where mental health is given as much priority as physical fitness in the pursuit of athletic excellence.

10.4 CULTURAL CONSIDERATIONS IN THE PRACTICE OF EFT

When introducing Emotional Freedom Techniques (EFT) into diverse cultural landscapes, we tread on a path that intertwines with deep-rooted beliefs, traditions, and communication styles. It's essential to approach this path with a high degree of respect and a willingness to adapt, ensuring that EFT is not perceived as an imposition but as a harmonious addition to existing cultural practices. One of the core strengths of EFT is its flexibility—its basic principles can be tailored to resonate with different cultural norms and values, making it a universally applicable tool for emotional and physical healing.

Cultural Sensitivity and Adaptation

Cultural sensitivity in EFT involves more than just understanding different customs or traditions; it requires an active integration of these elements into the practice of EFT to enhance its acceptance and effectiveness. For instance, in cultures where direct discussion of emotions is uncommon or taboo, EFT practitioners might focus more on physical symptoms and use gentle metaphors to address emotional issues indirectly. This approach respects and aligns with the cultural norms, fostering a more receptive environment for EFT. Additionally, incorporating culturally significant symbols or rituals into the tapping process can make the practice more relatable. For example, local idioms or culturally specific affirmations can help individuals connect more deeply with the EFT process, enhancing the therapeutic experience.

Language and Communication

The language used in EFT scripts plays a critical role in ensuring that the message resonates with the practitioner. This aspect becomes even more crucial when EFT is introduced to non-English speaking countries or diverse ethnic groups within broader communities. Offering translations of EFT scripts is a fundamental step, but ensuring that these translations are both linguistically accurate and culturally congruent is also necessary. Phrases and concepts used in EFT should be carefully adapted to maintain their effectiveness and reflect the users' cultural context. For instance, idiomatic expressions with positive connotations in one language might translate into something less impactful or confusing in another, potentially diluting EFT's effectiveness. Therefore, working with cultural consultants or bilingual practitioners to craft and review these scripts can significantly enhance their appropriateness and impact.

Case Studies from Different Cultures

The versatility of EFT is beautifully illustrated through its successful application across various cultural settings. Consider the case of a community project in a rural area of India where EFT was introduced to help women deal with stress and anxiety resulting from economic and social pressures. The facilitators adapted the EFT protocols to align with local practices, using local languages and culturally relevant metaphors that related to daily activities and traditional roles. The success of this project not only improved the well-being of the participants but also increased the community's openness to integrating EFT with other wellness practices. Another example can be seen in workshops conducted in urban Brazil, where EFT was used to help people cope with the stress of living in high-crime areas. Here, the sessions incorporated popular cultural elements like music and dance to help participants express their emotions more freely, enhancing the cathartic effect of EFT.

Training and Resources

For EFT practitioners working in culturally diverse environments, ongoing education and resources are vital to develop and maintain cultural competence. This training should include modules on cultural sensitivity, communication styles, and ethical considerations specific to different cultures, ensuring practitioners are well-prepared to adapt their methods appropriately. Additionally, resources like culturally adapted scripts, case studies, and guidelines for integrating EFT with local health practices can be invaluable. These resources support practitioners in delivering effective and respectful EFT sessions and contribute to EFT's broader acceptance and success in diverse settings.

As we conclude this exploration into the cultural considerations of EFT, it's clear that the true strength of this technique lies in its adaptability. By respecting and integrating cultural differences into the practice of EFT, practitioners can ensure that this powerful tool reaches its full potential in helping individuals across the globe manage stress, heal emotional pain, and achieve personal growth. The insights and strategies discussed here pave the way for EFT's more inclusive and practical application, highlighting its role as a bridge in the global community's pursuit of wellness and emotional resilience.

As we transition from this chapter into the broader aspects of EFT application in various life situations, it becomes evident that cultural sensitivity and adaptation principles are beneficial and essential for the holistic application of any therapeutic practice. This understanding enriches our approach, ensuring that as we move forward, we do so with a deep appreciation for the diverse tapestry of human experience that EFT serves.

CHAPTER 11
BEYOND TAPPING: COMPLEMENTARY PRACTICES

Imagine stepping into a serene space where every breath and movement brings you closer to an inner tranquility you thought was unattainable. Here, in this chapter, we explore how the gentle art of Emotional Freedom Techniques (EFT) can be beautifully woven together with meditation, a practice as ancient as it is profound. This fusion enhances the inherent soothing qualities of both techniques and elevates your journey to emotional clarity and calm. It's like mixing vibrant colors on a palette—separately they are captivating, but together they create something extraordinary.

11.1 COMBINING EFT WITH MEDITATION FOR ENHANCED CALM

Synergistic Effects of EFT and Meditation

The integration of EFT and meditation is akin to a dance between two harmonious forces, enhancing the other's ability to heal and soothe the mind. Each practice is powerful on its own, with EFT tapping into the body's energy system through meridian points and meditation, cultivating a state of deep peace and mindfulness. Combined, they amplify the calming effects, creating a dual pathway to relaxation and mental clarity. This synergy works because while EFT actively clears emotional blockages, meditation helps to stabilize these changes, embedding them deeper into your psyche. The result is a more profound and lasting shift towards emotional equilibrium and clarity of thought.

For those who battle with racing thoughts or chronic stress, this combination can be particularly transformative. EFT helps to surface and address unresolved emotional turmoil, while meditation fosters a newfound sense of peace and detachment from habitual stress responses. Together, they teach the mind and body a new way to react to old triggers, gradually rewiring years of conditioned responses to stress and anxiety.

Integrating Meditation Pre or Post-Tapping

Incorporating meditation into your EFT routine can be done with flexibility, depending on your personal needs and responses. Starting with a meditation session can prepare your mind, creating a fertile ground for the focused emotional work that tapping involves. It helps stabilize your mind, making you more receptive to acknowledging and processing the emotions that arise during tapping. On the other hand, ending your tapping session with meditation can help consolidate the emotional insights and shifts achieved during tapping. It allows you to absorb and extend the calmness and clarity elicited from your EFT practice.

Here's how you can seamlessly integrate these practices:

- Pre-Tapping Meditation: Begin with five minutes of focused breathing or guided meditation to calm your thoughts and mind. This preparation helps you approach EFT with a grounded and clear mindset, enhancing the effectiveness of your tapping session.
- Post-Tapping Meditation: After completing your EFT routine, transition into a meditative state by returning to your breath or engaging in a mindfulness exercise. This helps solidify any emotional shifts or resolutions from the tapping session, allowing the body and mind to integrate these changes fully.

Meditative Tapping Routines

Routines that incorporate both meditation and tapping can provide a structured way to enjoy the benefits of both practices. For instance, start with a brief meditation to center yourself, followed by EFT tapping on specific issues, and conclude with another meditation to reflect on the changes and stabilize your emotional state.

Here's a simple routine to get you started:

1. Begin with Mindful Breathing: Spend a few minutes in stillness, focusing solely on your breath. Let each inhale bring calm, and each exhale to release tension.
2. Engage in EFT: Tap through the points systematically, focusing on an issue you wish to address, using setup statements and reminder phrases that resonate with your current emotional state.

3. End with a Guided Meditation: Use a guided visualization to envision the resolution of your issue and feel the emotional relief and peace that comes with it.

Case Studies and Research

Studies have shown that such integrative approaches can significantly lower stress levels, improve emotional regulation, and enhance overall mental health. Empirical evidence supports the effectiveness of combining EFT with meditation. For example, a case study involving individuals with chronic anxiety reported marked improvements in anxiety levels and quality of life following a regimen that combined meditation and EFT, showcasing the potent effects of this dual approach.

In another documented instance, a group of high-stress professionals participated in a program that included EFT and mindfulness meditation. The results indicated not only a decrease in stress but also enhanced resilience and performance in their professional roles. These findings highlight the practical benefits of merging these practices into daily routines, providing a powerful toolkit for managing stress and fostering long-term emotional well-being.

Through the thoughtful integration of meditation and EFT, you can navigate the complexities of your emotions with greater ease and effectiveness. This chapter invites you to explore this synergy, encouraging you to weave these practices into your daily life, thus opening doors to deeper self-awareness, tranquility, and emotional freedom.

11.2 YOGA AND EFT: A SYMBIOTIC RELATIONSHIP FOR HEALING

Imagine enhancing your emotional freedom techniques (EFT) with yoga's physical grace and strength. This harmonious combination deepens your emotional release and fortifies your physical resilience, creating a holistic approach to wellness that resonates through every layer of your being. Yoga, with its rich tradition of promoting balance and flexibility, naturally complements the principles of EFT. As you engage in yoga, your body becomes more aligned, and your muscles stretch and strengthen, significantly enhancing energy flow during your tapping sessions. This physical alignment helps to clear the pathways, ensuring that the energy moves smoothly and effectively, thus amplifying the benefits of each tap.

Yoga positions, or asanas, target various meridian points that are also focal points in EFT. For instance, poses like Downward Dog and Cobra stretch and activate the spine where several meridians run, including the bladder and gallbladder meridians. Engaging in these poses before a tapping session can help awaken these energy pathways, making your EFT practice more dynamic and potent. Conversely, calming poses like Child's Pose target the heart and small intestine meridians, soothing and preparing your body for emotional work in EFT. This dual approach not only enhances the release of energy blockages but also supports a deeper emotional cleanse and restoration.

Creating a combined routine of yoga and EFT can initially seem daunting, but with a structured approach, it can quickly become a part of your daily wellness practice. Consider starting your morning with a few gentle yoga stretches to awaken the body and focus the mind. Simple poses that open up the chest and spine are particularly effective in preparing you for EFT. Transition into your EFT routine after your yoga session while your body is still supple and your mind calm. This could involve tapping into specific issues you've become aware of during your yoga practice. To end, you might return to a short yoga sequence, perhaps focusing on grounding poses like the Mountain or Tree pose, to consolidate the gains from your EFT session and stabilize your emotional state.

The stories of those who have integrated yoga and EFT into their healing journey are inspiring and instructive. Take, for example, Sarah, a middle-aged school teacher who battled chronic anxiety for years. Her introduction to EFT provided significant relief, but the integration of yoga into her tapping routines truly transformed her approach to stress. Each morning, Sarah began with a series of yoga poses that helped her feel more grounded and centered. She then moved into her EFT session, tapping on points already activated by her yoga practice. This combination not only enhanced her morning routine but also gave her practical tools to manage anxiety, leading to a noticeable improvement in her overall well-being and effectiveness at work.

Such stories underscore the practical applications and benefits of combining these powerful practices. They prove that aligning your body through yoga and clearing emotional blockages through EFT makes the path to wellness less arduous and more rewarding. Adopting these complementary practices enhances your ability to manage stress and emotional upheaval and invest in your long-term health and vitality, setting a foundation for a calmer, more centered existence.

11.3 USING VISUALIZATION TECHNIQUES ALONGSIDE TAPPING

Visualization is a powerful mental exercise that can significantly amplify the effectiveness of Emotional Freedom Techniques (EFT). When you visualize, you create detailed mental images of the desired outcomes or the emotional peace you wish to achieve. By integrating these vivid mental images with the physical act of tapping, you create a potent combination that can deeply imprint your intentions and accelerate your progress toward them. This process, known as enhancing imagery with tapping, involves focusing on specific visualizations while tapping on points that stimulate mental clarity and focus. For instance, while tapping on the forehead point, which is associated with insight and clarity, you might visualize yourself successfully achieving a personal goal, like delivering a flawless presentation or enjoying a peaceful family gathering. The tactile stimulation of the tapping points, combined with the mental imagery, helps to cement these positive visions in your subconscious, making them more attainable.

To effectively use visualization techniques alongside tapping, it is beneficial to develop scripts that incorporate detailed imagery. These scripts should guide you through a series of tapping points while prompting you to visualize specific scenarios that align with your emotional and psychological goals. For example, a script might begin with you tapping on the side of the hand (the karate chop point) while visualizing a barrier you face. As you continue tapping through the points on the face and body, the script would lead you through a scene where you see yourself overcoming this barrier easily and confidently. Each tapping point would focus on different aspects of the scenario, enhancing the emotional resonance of the visualization. This method helps reduce anxiety and stress and embeds a sense of capability and positivity regarding your ability to handle challenges.

Combining long-term goals with visualization and tapping is a strategic approach that aligns your daily practices with your broader aspirations. Suppose one of your long-term goals is to become more confident in social situations. In this case, you might use visualization to create detailed scenarios where you interact confidently with others. During each tapping session, focus on these visualizations, seeing yourself speaking clearly, making eye contact, and feeling relaxed in various social settings. By consistently tapping on these visualized outcomes, you reinforce the neural pathways associated with social confidence, gradually making these imagined behaviors your new reality. The sensory detail in your visualizations—such as the sound of your voice, the warmth of your smile, and the firmness of your handshake—further enriches the experience, making the practice more vivid and impactful.

Various tools and applications can benefit those looking to refine their visualization skills. Guided imagery tracks are an excellent resource; these audio recordings lead you through detailed visualizations, often accompanied by soothing background music that enhances relaxation and focus. Virtual reality (VR) applications offer an even more immersive visualization experience, allowing you to enter a three-dimensional environment that can be tailored to reflect your visualized goals. Simple audio prompts can also be effective, especially when they include affirmations or cues that reinforce your imagery work alongside your tapping sessions. These tools serve not only to enhance the quality of your visualizations but also to ensure that your practice remains engaging and aligned with your emotional healing and personal development goals.

By incorporating these visualization techniques into your EFT practice, you unlock a powerful synergy that accelerates emotional healing and personal growth. This integrated approach makes the tapping process more engaging and significantly enhances its effectiveness, helping you achieve a more profound sense of emotional well-being and closer alignment with your life goals. As you continue to explore and refine this combination of visualization and tapping, you may move more swiftly along the path to personal fulfillment and emotional freedom, equipped with tools that empower you to visualize and manifest the very best in your life.

11.4 THE ROLE OF NUTRITION IN ENHANCING EFT OUTCOMES

Understanding the interplay between what we eat and how we feel is crucial, especially when engaging in practices like Emotional Freedom Techniques (EFT) that aim to balance our emotional health. Nutrients from our diet affect neurotransmitter pathways, inflammation, and overall brain health, influencing our emotional state. For instance, omega-3 fatty acids found in fish like salmon and sardines are known for their anti-inflammatory properties and their role in brain health, impacting mood and emotional well-being. A deficiency in these essential fats can lead to mood swings and a decrease in cognitive function, potentially diminishing the effectiveness of EFT in achieving emotional balance. Similarly, complex carbohydrates found in whole grains help to increase the production of serotonin, a neurotransmitter that enhances mood and reduces stress. Integrating these nutrients into your diet can support and amplify the emotional benefits achieved through EFT by stabilizing mood and enhancing brain function.

Furthermore, foods that enhance energy flow and reduce inflammation can significantly complement the energy work done with EFT. Foods rich in antioxidants, such as berries, nuts, and green leafy vegetables, fight oxidative stress and inflammation in the body, promoting better energy flow through the meridians tapped during EFT sessions. These foods help clear the pathways, ensuring that energy moves freely, enhancing the healing process initiated by tapping. Incorporating such anti-inflammatory foods into your diet supports your physical health but also aids in maintaining the energetic balance needed for effective EFT practice.

When integrating nutritional changes with EFT, the approach should be gradual and mindful, ensuring these changes are sustainable and aligned with your overall health goals. Start by introducing one or two nutrient-rich foods into your diet each week, such as swapping a daily snack for a handful of nuts or adding a serving of vegetables to your meals. As you become more comfortable with these changes, gradually increase the variety and quantity of healthful foods. This slow integration helps your body to adjust without overwhelming it, making it easier to maintain these changes in the long run. Additionally, align these dietary adjustments with your EFT sessions by focusing your tapping on any resistance to change or feelings of deprivation that might arise. This can enhance your commitment to nurturing your body, making the dietary changes part of a holistic approach to health.

Several case studies have highlighted the impact of dietary changes in conjunction with EFT on overall health and wellness. For example, a study involving individuals with high-stress levels and poor nutritional habits introduced EFT and guidance on incorporating specific nutrients known to combat stress. Over several weeks, participants reported a reduction in stress and an increase in energy and overall well-being. Another case involved a person suffering from chronic fatigue who adopted an anti-inflammatory diet while regularly practicing EFT. The combination of dietary changes and EFT led to significant improvements in energy levels and reduced pain symptoms, illustrating how integrated approaches can enhance the quality of life.

Textual Element: Reflection Section

Reflect on your current dietary habits and how they might influence your emotional and physical health. Consider any changes you might implement to support your EFT practice and enhance its effectiveness. Write down a few minor dietary adjustments you can start this week and how you plan to integrate these changes with your EFT sessions.

In exploring the symbiotic relationship between nutrition and EFT, we've uncovered how the nutrients we consume can directly impact our emotional health and the efficacy of tapping. By understanding and implementing dietary choices that enhance energy flow, reduce inflammation, and support neurotransmitter function, you can significantly boost the outcomes of your EFT sessions. This holistic approach aligns with the goals of EFT and promotes a broader spectrum of health and wellness, paving the way for a more balanced and harmonious life.

As we conclude this chapter, remember that each step you take in integrating thoughtful nutrition and effective EFT practices brings you closer to achieving emotional equilibrium and a vibrant state of health. Let's carry forward this holistic perspective as we move into the next chapter, which will delve into strategies for maintaining these practices in the long term, ensuring that the benefits you gain are not fleeting but part of a sustained journey toward wellness.

CHAPTER 12

CONTINUING YOUR JOURNEY WITH EFT

Imagine you've just discovered a secret garden. As you step through the gate, you realize that each path offers a unique journey, each turn, a new perspective. This garden is much like your ongoing adventure with Emotional Freedom Techniques (EFT)—a landscape rich with opportunities for growth, healing, and discovery. As you continue to explore and deepen your understanding of EFT, you'll find that creating your own tapping scripts is akin to cultivating your own plots within this garden, tailored to your personal, emotional, and physical landscape.

12.1 DEVELOPING YOUR OWN TAPPING SCRIPTS

Understanding Script Fundamentals

At the heart of effective EFT practice lies the art of crafting personalized tapping scripts. These scripts are more than just words; they are structured expressions of your personal experiences and emotions designed to target specific issues. To construct a compelling script, start with framing the issue clearly. This involves identifying and articulating exactly what you are feeling or struggling with. It's crucial to be as specific as possible—vagueness can dilute the effectiveness of your tapping session.

Next, you'll need to construct a setup statement. This statement should acknowledge the issue and simultaneously affirm self-acceptance despite it. Typically beginning with "Even though I have this [issue], I deeply and completely accept myself," this statement sets the stage for a transformative EFT session. Following the setup, you create reminder phrases, which are short, concise phrases that you repeat while tapping on each point. These phrases keep you focused on the issue and reinforce the cognitive aspect of the tapping process.

Crafting these components carefully ensures that your tapping scripts are potent and resonant, directly addressing the roots of your emotional or physical challenges.

Personalization Techniques

Personalization is critical to maximizing the impact of your EFT scripts. Your emotions and experiences are uniquely yours; your scripts should reflect that individuality. Begin by reflecting deeply on how you experience your issue—what triggers it, what emotions are linked to it, and how it manifests in your life. This reflection helps tailor your setup statement and reminder phrases to your specific emotional reality.

Incorporating personal affirmations that resonate with your aspirations or self-perception can significantly enhance the power of your scripts. For instance, if confidence is an area you struggle with, embedding affirmations like "I am competent and strong" into your tapping routine can bolster your self-esteem over time.

Script Writing Exercises

To hone your script-writing skills, engage in regular exercises. Start with identifying a minor daily issue, perhaps procrastination or mild anxiety about public speaking. Write a specific setup statement for this issue, followed by reminder phrases. Tap through the script you've created, noting how it affects your emotional state.

Another effective exercise is to rewrite scripts for different emotions. Take a basic script and adapt it for sadness, anger, joy, or any other emotion you frequently encounter. This enhances your script-writing skills and deepens your emotional vocabulary, an essential component of effective EFT practice.

Feedback and Revision Strategies

Developing effective tapping scripts is an iterative process. After using a script, take time to reflect on its effectiveness. How did you feel before and after the session? Did specific phrases resonate more than others? Gathering this feedback through self—reflection or sharing your scripts with a trusted friend or therapist provides valuable insights that can guide script refinement.

Regularly revising your scripts based on this feedback ensures they remain aligned with your evolving emotional needs and continue to enhance their effectiveness. Much like tending to a garden, this feedback loop is crucial for growth and flourishing, helping refine your EFT techniques and deepen your healing journey.

In this ongoing process of script development, you become more adept at identifying and articulating your issues and enhancing your overall self-awareness and emotional intelligence. This personalized approach makes EFT more effective and a profoundly empowering tool fostering resilience, understanding, and profound emotional healing. As you continue to craft and refine your scripts, remember that each word and phrase is a step towards a more balanced and joyful self.

12.2 STAYING UPDATED: CONTINUING EDUCATION IN EFT

In the dynamic landscape of Emotional Freedom Techniques (EFT), staying updated with the latest advancements and deepening your understanding through continued education is essential for personal mastery and professional development. As you become more familiar with the critical practices in EFT, you might be eager to expand your knowledge and refine your skills. This can be achieved through a variety of resources designed for advanced learning. For instance, numerous books delve deeper into the nuances of EFT, offering insights into complex cases and specialized techniques. Titles such as "The Science of Tapping" by Dr. Peta Stapleton provide a solid foundation for the evidence-based approach to EFT, making complex information accessible and actionable.

Moreover, the digital age brings the convenience of online courses and workshops right to your fingertips. Platforms like Udemy, Coursera, and even specific EFT-focused sites offer sessions ranging from beginner to advanced levels, often led by renowned experts. These courses allow you to learn at your own pace and provide opportunities to interact with a global community of learners through forums and group discussions. Additionally, attending workshops and seminars offers a more hands-on approach to learning. These events are typically structured to provide live demonstrations, guided practice sessions, and direct feedback from experienced practitioners, enriching your learning experience and providing practical skills that can be immediately applied to your practice.

For those considering turning their passion for EFT into a professional career, becoming a certified EFT practitioner offers a pathway to enhance personal skills and gain credibility in the field. Certification programs, which various EFT organizations often offer, entail a comprehensive curriculum that covers advanced tapping techniques, client assessment skills, and ethical practices. The process usually culminates in an assessment that tests theoretical knowledge and practical application. The benefits of certification extend beyond personal satisfaction; it reassures clients of your commitment to quality and adherence to standardized practices, enhancing your professional reputation and expanding your career opportunities.

Keeping up with the latest research and developments in EFT is crucial for maintaining an evidence-based practice. This involves reading scientific studies and literature and participating in forums and conferences to discuss new ideas and findings. Subscribing to journals such as the "EFT International Journal" can provide updates on the latest research, case studies, and commentary from leading experts. Moreover, engaging with research enhances your understanding. It equips you with the knowledge to address skeptics of EFT with well-founded arguments and data, thereby advocating for the broader acceptance and application of EFT in various therapeutic contexts.

Engagement with professional EFT organizations is pivotal to your growth and development as a practitioner. These bodies offer resources for continued learning and a platform for networking with peers and mentors. Membership often comes with benefits such as access to exclusive seminars, discounted rates on conferences, and opportunities to contribute to newsletters or journals.

More importantly, these organizations uphold standards that ensure the integrity and effectiveness of EFT practices globally. By aligning yourself with these bodies, you commit to a standard of excellence and continuous improvement, ensuring that your practice remains relevant and contributes positively to the field of EFT.

As you navigate these resources and opportunities, remember that each step you take enhances your skills and contributes to the legitimacy and growth of EFT as a respected therapeutic practice. Whether through reading the latest publications, engaging in advanced courses, or participating actively in professional communities, your commitment to staying informed and educated transforms your practice. It enriches the collective understanding and application of EFT worldwide.

12.3 CONNECTING WITH THE EFT COMMUNITY: FINDING SUPPORT AND INSPIRATION

The vitality of any practice often stems not just from the knowledge and skills you accumulate but also from the connections you forge along your path. In Emotional Freedom Techniques (EFT), engaging with a community of fellow practitioners offers a tapestry of benefits that can enrich your personal and professional life. When you connect with others who share your passion for EFT, you tap into a wellspring of support, motivation, and inspiration. These connections can be particularly invaluable as they provide a network of encouragement, understanding, and empathy for the challenges and triumphs involved in practicing EFT.

Imagine walking into a room where everyone speaks your language of tapping points and emotional freedom. That's what it feels like to be part of an EFT community. Here, experiences and ideas flow freely, allowing you to glean new insights and share your own. This exchange can dramatically enhance your practice —learning how others handle particular emotional challenges or integrate unique techniques can open up new avenues for your own sessions. Moreover, the motivational boost from seeing others succeed and overcome similar hurdles can be incredibly uplifting, reaffirming your commitment to EFT and its benefits.

To begin weaving these vital connections, explore local and online EFT groups. Locally, you might find community centers, wellness clinics, or even private groups that hold regular meet-ups. Participating in these local groups supports your learning and embeds you within a network of practitioners nearby, making it easier to attend sessions and share experiences in person. Online, the world of EFT expands exponentially. Social media platforms, forums, and dedicated EFT websites host a plethora of groups where practitioners of all levels gather to discuss techniques, challenges, and breakthroughs. Platforms like Facebook and LinkedIn offer groups dedicated to EFT practice where you can post questions, share experiences, and connect with EFT experts globally.

The benefits of community engagement extend significantly when you actively participate in EFT events, workshops, and conferences. These gatherings are hubs of learning and connection, bringing together leading practitioners and enthusiasts worldwide. Workshops and conferences often feature sessions that allow you to refine your techniques under the guidance of EFT experts, participate in live demonstrations, and engage in discussions that deepen your understanding of complex aspects of EFT. Direct interaction bolsters your practical skills and provides a unique opportunity to network and build professional relationships that can lead to collaborations and growth opportunities.

Sharing your experiences within these communities is crucial in fostering a vibrant EFT culture. When you share your success stories or even the obstacles you've encountered, you contribute to a collective pool of knowledge that can help others navigate similar paths. This act of sharing can be profoundly gratifying—it's not just about giving back but also about validating your journey and the impact EFT has had on your life. Whether it's posting about a breakthrough you had with a client on an online forum or discussing a personal EFT experience at a conference, each story you share not only aids others but also enhances your own understanding and appreciation of the practice.

Therefore, engaging with the EFT community is not merely about networking or learning—it's about building a support system that encourages continuous personal and professional growth. It's about being part of a movement that celebrates emotional freedom and collective growth through shared experiences and mutual support. As you delve deeper into these communities, you find colleagues, friends, and mentors who can accompany you on your EFT adventure, making the journey all the more enriching and enjoyable. So, take the step, reach out, join a group, attend a workshop, share your story, and discover a community's profound impact on your EFT practice. This engagement propels your growth and contributes to the broader tapestry of Emotional Freedom Techniques, enriching it with your unique perspective and experiences.

12.4 THE FUTURE OF EFT: TRENDS AND INNOVATIONS

As we step into the future of Emotional Freedom Techniques (EFT), we witness a fascinating evolution of this therapeutic practice, characterized by its integration with diverse healing modalities and expansion into new demographic segments. Imagine a world where EFT is not just a standalone technique but part of an integrated therapy system, enhancing its effectiveness and appeal. Recently, there has been a significant trend toward combining EFT with cognitive-behavioral therapy (CBT), mindfulness-based stress reduction (MBSR), and even nutritional counseling, creating a more holistic approach to healing. This integration speaks to the versatility of EFT—it applies seamlessly with other therapies, enhancing outcomes by simultaneously addressing multiple dimensions of health.

Moreover, EFT is reaching a broader audience than ever before. Its simple, non-invasive nature makes it particularly appealing to diverse groups, including veterans dealing with PTSD, students facing academic stress, and even athletes looking to improve their mental game. Healthcare professionals are beginning to incorporate EFT into their practices, recognizing its potential to provide quick, effective relief from emotional distress. This trend towards inclusivity broadens the reach of EFT and enriches the practice with insights from a wide range of experiences and backgrounds, making it more adaptable and robust.

The influence of technology on EFT marks another exciting frontier. With the advent of smartphone apps and virtual reality (VR) systems, EFT is becoming more accessible. Apps designed to guide users through EFT sessions enable people to practice tapping anytime, anywhere, with just a few taps on their screen. These apps often include customizable scripts, reminders, and tracking systems to monitor progress, making self-led EFT practice more accessible and practical. Additionally, virtual reality offers an immersive way to practice EFT by placing users in controlled, calming environments that enhance the tapping experience. Imagine donning a VR headset and being transported to a tranquil beach or a quiet forest where you can practice EFT without distractions—this could be a regular practice in the near future.

Predictions for the evolution of EFT suggest a continued expansion of its applications and methodologies. Experts anticipate that future developments will include more precise ways to measure the physiological effects of tapping, such as real-time monitoring of brain activity and hormonal responses. This could lead to more personalized EFT protocols tailored to individuals' specific physiological patterns, enhancing the therapy's effectiveness. Furthermore, as our understanding of the genetic basis of emotion and behavior grows, there might be opportunities to integrate EFT with genetic counseling, providing interventions customized to psychological and physical needs and genetic predispositions.

Staying ahead of these changes requires a proactive approach. For those keen on keeping your EFT practice current and practical, staying informed about the latest technological advancements and research findings is crucial. Engaging with online platforms that offer continuous learning opportunities, subscribing to journals that focus on EFT research, and participating in forums where innovations are discussed are excellent ways to keep your finger on the pulse of emerging trends. Furthermore, experimenting with new tools and techniques, such as incorporating app-based EFT into your sessions or exploring VR environments, can enhance your practice and provide you with firsthand insights into the practical applications of these innovations.

As the landscape of EFT continues to evolve, embracing these trends and innovations will ensure that your practice remains relevant and practical. The future of EFT is vibrant and promising, with endless possibilities for growth, learning, and healing. By staying informed, adaptable, and open to new ideas, you can continue to harness the full potential of EFT, helping both yourself and others achieve greater emotional freedom and well-being.

In summary, we've explored the dynamic future of EFT, from its integration with various therapeutic modalities and expansion into new demographic areas to the exciting technological advancements enhancing its accessibility and effectiveness. As we close this chapter on the future trends and innovations in EFT, let's carry forward the spirit of curiosity and openness, ready to explore new horizons and embrace the evolving landscape of emotional health and wellness.

UNLOCK THE POWER OF GENEROSITY

"One of the most beautiful ways to lift ourselves is by lifting others."

— UNKNOWN

Thank you for reading *Tapping Into Freedom* by Eloise Rose. Your journey through this book has shown you the simple yet powerful effects of tapping. By taking just a few minutes to share your thoughts, you can help others discover this tool for themselves.

Leaving a review is as simple as sharing your experience. Did Tapping Into Freedom show you a new way to calm your mind or ease your worries? Did it make you feel more at peace? Did it help you or someone you care about? Share that! Your experience can be the light that guides someone else, whether big or small.

Your review doesn't have to be long. A few sentences can go a long way in helping others see the value of tapping and how this book can be a helpful guide.

Scan to leave a review!

Thank you for your generosity and for being a part of this journey. Your contribution is invaluable. Just tap on the link below to share your experience and help others on their path to freedom.

With gratitude,
Eloise Rose

CONCLUSION

As we reach the final pages of this journey together, I want to reflect on the path we've traversed. You've shown remarkable dedication, from the first steps of understanding the basics of Emotional Freedom Techniques (EFT) to mastering sophisticated tapping strategies for various emotional and physical issues. Your willingness to explore and integrate EFT into your life is commendable; it's a powerful testament to your commitment to personal well-being and growth.

Throughout this book, we've delved into the foundational aspects of EFT, uncovering its roots and the science that supports its efficacy. You've learned how to set up tapping sessions, handle emotional upheavals gracefully, and apply tapping to physical symptoms, stress, and anxiety. More importantly, we've seen how EFT serves as a tool for momentary relief and a profound method for deep emotional and physical healing.

The key takeaway from our time together is the transformative power of EFT. This technique is not just about coping with life's challenges; it's about opening doors to personal transformation and long-lasting wellness. Tapping offers a pathway to heal past traumas, enhance self-confidence, and foster a resilient spirit, making it a versatile and accessible method for anyone committed to holistic health.

Now, I encourage you to continue your journey with EFT. The effectiveness of tapping grows with regular practice. Engage with the EFT community, share your experiences, and continue learning. Every tap and session adds depth to your understanding and strengthens your ability to handle whatever life throws your way.

Thank you for allowing me to guide you through the fantastic world of EFT. Your role in spreading the knowledge and benefits of this powerful healing tool is invaluable. By sharing your success and insights, you contribute to your health and the well-being of others around you.

Let's conclude with a note of inspiration: Embrace EFT as a lifelong companion on your journey toward healing, growth, and fulfillment. Remember, the journey with EFT is just beginning. The possibilities for transformation are limitless, and the potential for personal freedom and empowerment is immense.

EFT is more than just a technique; it's a journey toward personal freedom, healing, and empowerment. Embrace this journey with your heart and mind open, ready to explore the depths of your own healing potential. Here's to moving forward with confidence, equipped with a powerful tool that promises relief and a pathway to a more vibrant, fulfilled life.

REFERENCES

Ambler, H. (2017). 3 powerful ways to use EFT tapping to achieve your goals. *Heather Ambler* https://www.heatherambler.com/single-post/2017/01/01/3-powerful-ways-to-use-tapping-to-achieve-your-goals-1

Ambler, H. (n.d.). Tapping for Grief. How to use EFT to recover from loss. *Heather Ambler*. https://www.heatherambler.com/single-post/efttappingforgrief

Church, D. (2018). Guidelines for the treatment of PTSD using clinical EFT. *Journal of Clinical Psychology. 74*(6), 1070-1082. https://www.ncbi,nih,gov/pmc/articles/PMC6316206/

Church, D., & Brooks, A.J. (2022). Clinical EFT as an evidence-based practice for The treatment of psychological and physiological conditions. *Journal Of Evidence-Based Integrative Medicine, 27*. https://pubmed.ncbi.nlm.nih.gov/36438382/

Church, D., & Stapleton, P. (2019). Clinical EFT (Emotional Freedom Techniques) Improves multiple physiological markers of health. *Journal of Evidence-Based Integrative Medicine, 24*. https://www.ncbi.nlm.nih.gov/pmc/articles/PMC6381429/

Chilton, L. (n.d.). How to use positive tapping affirmations for confidence. *Calmpreneur*. https://calmpreneur.com/positive-tapping-affirmations-confidence-eft/

Clond, M. (2016). EFT tapping: The psychology behind tapping therapy. *Positive Psychology*. https://positivepsychology.com/eft-tapping/

Craig, G. (n.d.). How to design your own EFT setup phrases. *EFT Universe*. https://eftuniverse.com/refinemets-to-eft/creating-custom-designed-eft-setup-phrases/

Feinstein, D. (n.d.). 10 top misconceptions about EFT. *EFT Universe*. https://eftuniverse.com/10-top-misconceptions-about-eft/

Gallo, F. (n.d.). The origin and history of EFT - Emotional Freedom Techniques. *EFT Help*. https://www.eft-help.com/intro/EFThistory.htm

Gallo, F. (n.d.) EFT tapping success stories & testimonials. *EFT Universe*. https://eftuniverse.com/stories/

Jacobs, J. (n.d.). Releasing the fear from within with EFT. *EFT International*. https://eftinternatonal.org/releasing-the-fear-from-within-with-eft/

Lane, J.R. (2023). Emotional freedom techniques (EFT). Tap to relieve stress and

154 REFERENCES

Anxiety. *Journal of Nervous and Mental Disease, 211*(1), 44-52. https://www.ncbi.nlm.nih.goc/pmc/articles/PMC9840127/

Ortner, J. (n.d.). EFT tapping for sleep: Could this be the breakthrough solution to your sleep problems? The Tapping Solution. https://www.thetappingsolution.com/blog/eft-tapping-for-sleep-could-this-be-the-breakthrough-solution-to-your-sleep-problems/

Ortner, J. (n.d.). Tapping 101 – Learn the basics of the tapping technique. *The Tapping Solution*. https://www.thetappingsolution.com/tapping-101/

Ortner, N. (n.d.). Community tapping circle - Join us free, live. *EFT Universe*. https://eftuniverse.com/community-tapping-circle/

Ortner, N. (n.d.). EFT tapping chart: Getting to know the 9 tapping points. *The Tapping Solution*. https://www.thetappingsolution.com/blog/eft-tapping-chart-getting-to-know-the-9-main-tapping-points/

Ortner, N. (n.d.). How to use EFT tapping to help reduce pain. *The Tapping Solution*. https://www.thetappingsolution.com/blog/how-to-use-tapping-pain-relief/

Ortner, N. (n.d.). Start your morning with this 5-minute tapping ritual. *Life Goals Magazine*. https://lifegoalsmag.com/start-your-morning-with-this-5-minute-tapping-ritual/

Ortner, N. (n.d.). The top 5 mistakes people make with EFT tapping and how to correct them. *The Tapping Solution*. https://www.thetappingsolution.com/blog/the-top-5-mistakes-people-make-with-eft-tapping-and-how-to-correct-them/

Ortner, N. (n.d.). Tapping for depression: Unlocking the benefits of EFT. *The Tapping Solution*. https://www.thetappingsolution.com/blog/unlocking-the-benefits-of-tapping-for-depression/

Ortner, J. (n.d.). What mindfulness meditation and EFT tapping have in common. *The Tapping Solution*. https://www.thetappingsolution.com/blog/what-mindfulness-meditation-and-eft-have-in-common/

Patton, D. (n.d.). EFT tapping for panic attacks: A holistic approach. *Vitality Living College*. https://vitalitylivingcollege.info/eft-tapping-for-panic-attacks-a-holistic-approach/

Patton, D. (n.d.). How to cope with workplace stress with EFT tapping? *Vitality Living College*. https://vitalitylivingcollege.info/how-to-cope-with-stress-in-the-workplace-with-eft-apping/

Patton, D. (n.d.). How does EFT tapping help in setting and achieving goals? Vitality Living College. https://vitalitylivingcollege.info/how-does-eft-tapping-help-in-setting-and-achieving-goals/

Patton, D. (n.d.). Tapping for relationship issues: Emotional healing. *Vitality

Living College*. https://vitalitylivingcollege.info/eft-tapping-for-relationship-issues/

Poole, H. (2024). Effectiveness and feasibility of structured emotionally focused therapy. *Journal of Clinical Psychology, 80*(4), 333-340. https://www.ncbi.nlm.nih.gov/pmc/articles/PMC10289383/

Rees, A. (n.d.). Learn how seniors can benefit from EFT tapping. *PARC Living*. https://parcliving.ca/blog/learn-how-seniors-can-benefit-from-eft-tapping/

Tapper, M. (n.d.). Four EFT tapping success stories spread the word about EFT. *EFT Universe*. https://eftuniverse.com/insomnia/four-eft-tapping-success-stories-spread-the-word-about-eft/

Tapping Solution. (n.d.). EFT to resolve anger issues - A case study approach. *International Journal of Holistic Wellness, 10*(2), 55-70. Retrieved August 20, 2024, from https://www.researchgate.net/publication/377444609_EFT_to_Resolve_Anger_Issues_-_A_Case_Study_Approach_IJHW_June_2022

Woo, L. (n.d.) *Unlocking Emotional Freedom: Utilizing EFT for Phobias*. Quenza https://quenza.com/blog/knowledge-base/eft-for-dealing-with-phobias/

Made in the USA
Columbia, SC
18 January 2025

c0b6aff1-1e68-498a-af2d-1d334caad0caR01